OXFORD HANDBOOKS IN EMERGENCY MEDICINE
Series Editors R. N. Illingworth, C. E. Robertson, and A. D. Redmond

D1635857

OXFORD HANDBOOKS IN EMERGENCY MEDICINE

This series covers topics of interest to all Accident and Emergency staff. The books are aimed at junior doctors and casualty nurses. Each book starts with an introduction to the topic, including epidemiology where appropriate. The clinical presentation and the immediate practical management of common conditions is described in detail, so that the casualty officer or nurse is able to deal with the problem on the spot. A specific course of action is recommended for each situation, and alternatives discussed.

History Taking, Examination, and Record Keeping in Emergency Medicine

H. R. Guly
Consultant, Accident and Emergency Medicine,
Derriford Hospital, Plymouth

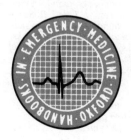

Oxford • New York • Tokyo
OXFORD UNIVERSITY PRESS
1996

Oxford University Press, Walton Street, Oxford OX2 6DP

Oxford   New York
Athens   Auckland   Bangkok   Bombay
Calcutta   Cape Town   Dar es Salaam   Delhi
Florence   Hong Kong   Istanbul   Karachi
Kuala Lumpur   Madras   Madrid   Melbourne
Mexico City   Nairobi   Paris   Singapore
Taipei   Tokyo   Toronto
and associated companies in
Berlin   Ibadan

Oxford is a trade mark of Oxford University Press

Published in the United States
by Oxford University Press Inc., New York

A catalogue record for this book is available from the British Library

Library of Congress Cataloging in Publication Data

Guly, H. R. (Henry R.)
History taking, examination, and record keeping in emergency
medicine/H.R. Guly.
p. cm. — (Oxford handbooks in emergency medicine; 12)
Includes bibliographical references and index.
1. Communication in emergency medicine — Handbooks, manuals, etc.
2. Medical history taking — Handbooks, manuals, etc.   I. Title.   II. Series.
[DNLM: 1. Medical History Taking — methods — handbooks.   2. Physical
Examination — methods — handbooks.   3. Medical Records — handbooks.
4. Emergency Medicine — methods — handbooks.   WB 39 098 v. 12 1996]
RC86.3.G85   1995   616.07'51 — dc20   DNLM/DLC
for Library of Congress   95-20108 CIP
ISBN 0-19-262462-8 (hbk: alk. paper). — ISBN 0-19-262461-X (pbk: alk. paper)

Typeset by Footnote Graphics, Warminster, Wiltshire
Printed in Great Britain on acid-free paper by
Biddles Ltd, Guildford & King's Lynn

To Maeve

Contents

PART 1

General considerations

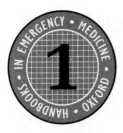

CHAPTER 1

Introduction

Skill in the arts of history taking, physical examination and record keeping is essential for good medical care. Although taught at length at medical school, pressures on the curriculum may mean that not enough emphasis is given to trauma and other musculoskeletal problems. Preregistration house officer appointments are usually in general medicine and surgery and therefore many 'casualty officers' begin their work in accident and emergency with little knowledge of trauma and musculoskeletal problems. Add to this the facts that many A&E departments are very busy with doctors under great pressure to see patients quickly and the record cards are frequently small with little room to write, it is not surprising that A&E records are frequently very poorly completed. In every branch of medicine good records are essential and this is particularly true in A&E with its numerous medicolegal problems and the frequent need to produce records for evidence in legal cases.

This book aims to guide newly appointed casualty officers, and any other doctor who treats similar problems (e.g. in general practice or in industry), on how keep adequate records on the conditions they will see and treat. In A&E, doctors and nurses work together as a team more closely than in many other specialties and nurses will frequently record their notes on the A&E record card. I am grateful therefore to Mrs Annie Jenkins for her chapter on nursing records. Increasingly nurses, who have never before been taught diagnostic skills, are taking on a nurse practitioner role in A&E departments and I hope that the rest of this book may guide them also. In order to record good information it is necessary first to obtain it. Therefore the essential elements of history and examination are included for each type of injury and every part of the body. It is sometimes argued that there is not enough time to write proper notes and that it is more important to treat patients. This is a false argument. Poor note keeping usually reflects poor clinical method. It is also a dangerous argument as will be demonstrated in the next chapter.

The medical defence organizations constantly stress the importance of good records.[1,2] Good, well-thought out notes do not take long to write and to prove this I give examples of adequate (although not necessarily perfect) records in each chapter. Every consultant will have his or her own preferences on what notes should contain and if they have a particular clinical or research interest or 'bee in their bonnet' they may wish more information to be gathered than I recommend. However, if all A&E records were kept along the lines put forward in this book there would be enormous benefits to both patients and doctors.

References

1. Hill, G. (1991). *A&E risk management*. Medical Defence Union, London.
2. MDU (Medical Defence Union) (1992). *Medical records*. Medical Defence Union. London.

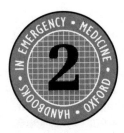

CHAPTER 2

Reasons for note keeping

Key points in note keeping
- Poor records = poor medicine.
- If it's not written down, it wasn't done.

There are four main reasons why it is important to keep notes.

1. To remind the doctor of details of the consultation. The patient will often be asked to return for review or may re-attend without an appointment if their symptoms become worse. Many patients need reports written for an employer, the police or an insurance company. A doctor seeing 40 patients a shift, will find it impossible to remember details of every patient even a week later, let alone the following year, but, not infrequently, if shown the notes of a patient seen several years earlier, will be able to remember much about the patient, the injury, and the consultation.

2. If a patient returns later and sees another doctor, the notes made at the original visit will indicate what was found, thought, done, and said. This is clearly important as it avoids unnecessary repetition of the history, examination, and investigations and allows a management plan to be followed. It is important that notes are as precise as possible. A note which says 'erythema left thigh' may or may not be helpful but to write 'erythema left thigh 15 × 12 cm' gives a measurement against which improvement or deterioration can be judged.

3. The notes which a doctor makes at the time are assumed, in law, (unless there is evidence to the contrary), to be an accurate record of what was found and what actually occurred at the consultation. This is important from the patient's point of view because if the patient sustains an injury and wishes to bring a civil lawsuit against the person responsible, or if the police wish to charge the patient's assailant, the A&E records are a legal document which may be produced to support a victim's case. The same notes are frequently of great value if a complaint is made, or a legal case brought, against the doctor. If there is a complaint that the doctor failed to examine adequately the patient or failed to warn of a side-effect of some drug, etc., the notes will be looked at and what is written in them will be assumed to have occurred. If the notes are comprehensive and legible then frequently a brief inspection will indicate immediately that there is no evidence of negligence even if there has, perhaps, been an error of judgement. On the other hand, if a patient returns to an A&E department with an obvious tendon injury 10 days after a laceration, a set of notes which reads 'laceration wrist, clean and suture' will make any claim of negligence indefensible as there is no evidence that tendon (or nerve) function has been examined. A plea that one always tests tendon function or even that one remembers testing it will be of little avail if the patient denies it was examined. The patient's evidence will probably be preferred as it will be assumed that the patient who only attends the A&E department infrequently will have a better memory of the event than the doctor who sees many patients every day. What is not written down may be assumed not to have happened.

As notes are a legal document, it follows that they must never be altered. Notes can never record every detail of the consultation and so it is possible that if the doctor later discovers that an error was made (or if a complaint is made), they can remember more details of what was said and done.

Details of these can be added but a line should be drawn under the previous entry in the notes and the new notes should be prefaced by a statement such as: 'the following notes were added on (date) at (time)'.

4. The information in the notes may be useful for research and audit. As good clinical care demands good notes, the quality of medical notes themselves is frequently a subject of audit.

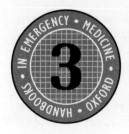

CHAPTER 3

Basic pattern of notes

Key points in basic pattern of notes
- Every entry in the notes should be dated and timed.
- Never abbreviate left and right.
- Notes must be legible.
- Write your name in capital letters under your signature.

Times

Every patient contact should be dated and the time noted to give a chronological record of the care given. Even for a relatively minor problem the notes might record:

- Time patient books in.
- Time seen by triage nurse.
- Time first seen by doctor.
- Time patient returns from X-ray.
- Time wounds are sutured.
- Time patient leaves the department.

The time a patient waits to be seen or waits on a trolley before admission is a measure of quality of care and it should be possible to identify these times for each patient. Accurate times are clearly important if a patient makes a complaint of having to wait an excessive length of time. Timings are also important for audit, planning, and the generation of statistics. Accurate waiting time statistics are becoming essential to satisfy the purchasers of A&E services, that agreed standards are being achieved. Many departments have computerized record systems and accurate timings mean that 'mean waiting times' or 'total time in the department' can be calculated. Times are more important for specific clinical problems. For a patient with a myocardial infarction, the time it takes from entering hospital to reaching the coronary care unit or to getting thrombolysis is a measure of quality and should be audited. Similarly, in patients with a dislocation of the hip, the risk of avascular necrosis is related to the time before it is reduced. A record of the time of the reduction may assist the orthopaedic surgeon in giving an accurate prognosis.

Legibility

It should go without saying that notes must be legible. Not only must other doctors be able to read medical notes but increasingly, doctors' handwriting has to be read and transcribed into computers by clerks who have had no medical training and who will not be able to interpret words from the context. Nonsensical information entered into computers not only causes problems with the generation of statistics but computerized information is used to generate letters to the general practitioner, discharge summaries etc. which will be worthless if based on incorrect data. A&E records may also be used to generate prescriptions. If a patient is given the wrong medication because of poor handwriting, the doctor is liable.

Abbreviations

Particular care must be taken when describing which side of the body has been injured and the words 'left' and 'right' must never be abbreviated. Unfortunately, mistakes are sometimes made and even when the side is correctly identified, L and R, when written quickly, can both end up looking like ℓ. It is not uncommon for the wrong limb to be X-rayed and operations on the wrong side are not unknown.

Abbreviations can be used in the notes as long as they are standard and would be understood country-wide and not just in the hospital where the patient is being seen. They should not be used in letters to general practitioners or to doctors in other specialties who may not understand the abbreviations used or who may use the same abbreviation to describe another disease. The general practitioner who received a letter containing the following lines wrote to demand a translation:

'**Diagnosis**: STI MCs
Treatment: Crepe, R/V GP PRN'

(Diagnosis: soft tissue injury to metacarpals. Treatment: crepe bandage, advised to return to general practitioner if required.)

Arrangement of notes

Notes should have the following arrangement:

- History.
- Examination.
  (provisional or differential diagnosis)
  (X-rays or other investigations performed)
  (results of X-rays or other investigations)
- Final diagnosis.
- Treatment.
- Advice to patient.
- Follow-up arrangements.
- Signature.

In addition details of essential telephone calls should be recorded. Imprecise statements such as: 'Discussed with orthopaedic registrar' should be avoided. All four of them may later forget or deny the conversation took place but a note stating 'Discussed with Mr X' cannot be misunderstood.

A senior doctor asked to give an opinion on a patient must repeat essential parts of the history and examination and establish that the notes recorded by a junior colleague are accurate. There is no need to record them again other than to say e.g. 'History and examination as above' but they should record their own decision making e.g. 'Agree X-rays show NBI'.

Signature

It is important that every person (doctor, nurse, medical student, paramedic, social worker etc.) who assesses the patient or carries out any practical procedure can be identified by a signature. This is because it may be necessary to identify the people who saw a particular patient several years after the event (by which time the head of department will certainly not recognize most signatures and may even have forgotten the junior doctor!). It is important that this signature is legible. Those doctors with traditionally illegible signatures should either write their names in capital letters after their signature or have a rubber stamp made of their name. Students' notes must, of course, be countersigned by a qualified person who will take responsibility for them. When patients are managed by a team, everyone must be identified. Ideally, each should write down their own involvement in the case and sign it but where this does not happen, the person compiling the notes should list all those involved.

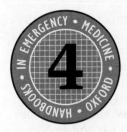

CHAPTER 4

Medical history

Key points in medical history
- Understanding the mechanism of injury is vital.
- The past medical history will often influence the patient's management.

The main aim of taking a history from a patient is to establish a diagnosis and to ensure that there are no factors in the past medical history which would interfere with treatment. There are also other aims which may be as important. Treatment, and certainly the explanation of the injury and the advice which one gives to a patient will usually need to be individualized depending on the patient's age, occupation, interests, intelligence, etc. In injuries of the upper limb it is important to know if the injury is to the dominant or non-dominant side. Talking more widely to the patient while taking the history will establish a relationship allowing one to get to know them. A doctor or nurse may need a different explanation of their injury than a patient who knows no anatomy or physiology and a musician will need enormous reassurance about any hand injury. Many fears of long-term disability etc. will be unspoken and so the doctor must be sensitive to hidden tensions and if necessary ask if the patient has any specific worries. Establishing a relationship with a patient (even if only for three minutes) will benefit patient care and improve patient (and doctor) satisfaction. Relevant information must be recorded.

The history of an injury should always contain the following information:

- When did it happen?
- Mechanism of injury?
- How (and why) did it happen?
- What happened next?
- Any significant past medical history?

Sometimes the history will also need to contain:

- Where it happened.
- Who was involved.

When did it happen?

If a patient presents to an emergency department, it is easy to fall into the trap of assuming their problem is acute. It may be of long-standing or an acute exacerbation of a chronic problem. When the injury occurred must always be recorded but notes such as 'Fell on Thursday' will mean nothing when read some weeks later. Either write down how many days previously the problem started or state the date. Do not mix these two methods; write either:

'23.6 stood on nail
24.6 foot became slightly red and painful
25.6 very painful, unable to weight bear, painful lumps in
       groin'

or

'3/7 ago stood on nail
2/7   foot became slightly red and painful
1/7   very painful . . .'

not

'Thursday last stood on nail
23.6   foot became slightly red and painful
1/7 ago   very painful . . .'

Mechanism of injury

It is of vital importance to understand the forces involved as this may give valuable clues to the diagnosis. High velocity impacts will cause a different pattern of injuries than low velocity impacts. The exact mechanism of injury may also be very important in establishing a diagnosis. For example in the ankle, an inversion injury may cause a sprain or a lateral malleollar fracture but a fall on to the heel may cause a calcaneal fracture. An acute pain behind the ankle, which occurs while running, is a 'classical' account of a ruptured Achilles tendon. A hand laceration caused by a sharp knife should be assumed to have divided tendons or nerves until proved otherwise but a similar looking wound caused by a blunt force is likely to cause an underlying fracture. A wound caused by broken glass may divide tendons and nerves and leave foreign bodies in the wound. A history of injury which reads 'Cut hand', 'Ankle injury' or 'RTA' is totally inadequate. Always ask 'What happened?' and ask further questions until you are sure in your own mind of the sequence of events. This history should be recorded using the patient's own words if possible and when used they should be put in quotation marks. This is not always possible as patients use gestures and movements to explain the method of injury but rather than writing:

'Valgus strain right knee'

it is better to write:

'Walking and left leg went into a hole, right knee stressed, tibia appeared to go laterally'

If a patient has fallen, record:

• How far they have fallen.
• What the patient landed on (e.g. concrete, earth).
• How the patient landed.

Patients do not always tell the truth about the mechanism of injury and if the findings on clinical examination do not correspond to the mechanism of injury, it is important to ask the patient to confirm the history. For example, if a patient presents with a laceration over the 4th metacarpophalangeal joint, the most likely explanation is that he has been fighting and has caught his hand on an opponent's teeth. This is a potentially very serious injury with the possibility of developing a septic arthritis of the joint. Clearly other mechanisms of injury are possible but as the treatment of a human bite injury is so different from that of a simple laceration, it is necessary to confront the patient with your suspicions and if necessary make a note such as:

'Cut hand on a corned beef tin—denies fighting'

If a child's injuries are not consistent with the stated mechanism the possibility of child abuse must be considered. In this case write down the stated history as fully as possible. The first account given may be very important if the parents change their story later but it should be left to a more senior doctor to question the parents further.

How (and why) did it happen?

How and why injuries occur normally becomes obvious when asking about the mechanism of injury and if the reason for the accident is not volunteered, normal curiosity will usually make the doctor ask. It is important that this question is answered as the reason for the injury may be more important than the injury itself. An old person who falls may have tripped but it is important to ensure that the fall was not caused by a cardiac arrhythmia, postural hypotension, a transient cerebral ischaemic attack, or some other cause. At the other end of the age spectrum it is important to ensure that a child's accident is not the result of neglect or abuse. In all age groups, by asking how and why accidents occur, A&E staff are ideally placed to identify dangerous road junctions or playground equipment etc., to point out home hazards to individual patients and to make recommendations for safe practice to local industry and the providers of leisure facilities.

Alcohol intoxication is a common cause of accidents and

where this has played a role, it should be noted. A&E departments are ideally placed to detect alcohol-related problems
of many sorts and, if the patient wants to be helped, to advise
the patient or to refer them for help. An alcohol-induced
injury presenting to A&E should therefore lead to some
further enquiries about consumption and the the effect it is
having on the patient, e.g.

'4 pints/night = 56 units/week. Occasional (6 or 7 × per year)
binges of up to 15 pints and spirits. Admits he has a problem. Advised to go to psychiatric crisis service tomorrow.
GP informed'

What happened next?

A knowledge of what happened after the injury may give
valuable clues to the diagnosis. A footballer who injured his
knee and continued to play is highly unlikely to have a
significant injury and a patient with a normal-looking hand
may have had a dislocation of the finger which they reduced
themselves. It is also important to discover what treatment
the patient may have already had from their general practitioner or anyone else.

Any significant past medical history?

In all but the most trivial injuries, a knowledge of the past
history is important. This may be important for diagnosis.
For example, the rigid cervical spine of ankylosing spondylitis may fracture with minimal trauma as may the spine
with a metastatic deposit and the anticoagulated patient who
has a head injury is at risk of an intracranial haematoma. A
past history of previous injury or coincidental disease may
be important when interpreting X-rays and a whole variety
of medical problems, medications, and allergies may affect
patient management in many ways. Although an anaesthetist
should always assess an injured patient before anaesthesia
it is the responsibility of the A&E department to discover
and draw to the anaesthetist's attention any obvious prob-

lems. For non-traumatic problems the past history is even more important: many an excised 'sebaceous cyst' has been reported histologically as a metastasis and even if a new symptom is not related to some previous significant illness knowledge of the previous problem will enable the doctor to reassure the patient whose unspoken fear is that the two are connected. Other aspects of the past medical history such that the patient is deaf and lip reads or that they have learning difficulties or are normally confined to a wheelchair are clearly of relevance and must be noted.

Where did the injury occur?

This may occasionally be of relevance: if a dog bite occurred in Great Britain, the possibility of rabies at present can be ignored but it may need to be considered in those whose injury occurred abroad.

Who was involved?

Whenever a history is obtained from someone other than the patient, it is important to record from whom it was obtained. This enables the history to be checked. A witness to an accident will give a more accurate account than a relative who has been told about it but a close relative will usually know more about the past medical history and medication than a neighbour. If an ambulance person gives details of the accident or the patient's past medical history, it is important to ask (and record) from whom they obtained the information. For assault victims it may be important to record who the assailant is alleged to be and, if a child is brought to A&E by anyone other than a parent, record who has brought them (e.g. teacher, grandparent).

Direct questioning

Following an injury it is important to know what symptoms the patient has. If the patient is uncommunicative they may not volunteer any symptoms and so will need to be asked direct questions but this will usually give less information than allowing the patient to give a history in their own words. As in other branches of medicine, a presenting symptom may suggest a possible diagnosis or differential diagnosis and questions may need to be answered to elucidate this. If these are not volunteered by the patient they will need to be asked as straight questions. For example, a patient with knee pain following an injury should be asked whether they have symptoms such as locking, catching, or giving way of the knee which might suggest a mechanical cause for the knee pain.

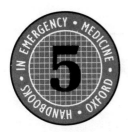

CHAPTER 5

Pain

Pain, of various sorts, is the commonest presenting symptom in A&E departments and in many other medical specialties. Adequate pain relief must be sought, not just for humanitarian reasons but because pain has adverse effects on the cardiovascular, respiratory, and neuroendocrine systems. Also, from the practical point of view, the patient in pain is anxious and difficult to manage. If pain is to be adequately controlled its severity before and after analgesia must be measured in some way. The simplest way of doing this is to ask patients to rate their pain none/mild/moderate/severe. An alternative and probably better way of assessing the severity of pain is the use of a visual analogue scale. A patient indicates the severity of their pain by making a mark on a 10 cm line whose ends represent no pain and the worst pain they can imagine (Fig. 5.1). Every patient in pain must be asked 'How bad is the pain?' and some will certainly benefit from proper measurement. A patient with a longer-standing problem should be asked what analgesics they have already tried and what effect they had.

No   Worst pain
pain   imaginable

Fig. 5.1 • A 10 cm analogue scale for measuring pain.

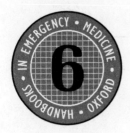

CHAPTER 6

Examination

In many branches of medicine physical examination of a patient may concentrate on the symptomatic area but will involve an examination of the whole body. In A&E, examination will usually be more restricted and the aim of this book is to state what examination should be performed for each part of the body. One of the important reasons for junior doctors working in A&E is to learn and practise the skills of examination of the musculoskeletal system and to learn to differentiate the normal from the pathological at all ages. Many injuries are missed because a doctor takes shortcuts in the history and examination and so once learned, this examination should be done **every time**. With practice, a full examination of any part of the body can be done efficiently and speedily.

Physical examination of a patient is also important as a means of establishing a relationship with the patient which a doctor needs in order to explain the disease and reassure the patient. When patients attend a doctor they expect to be physically examined and will be unhappy if they are not. Every doctor has heard a patient explain about a previous contact with the medical profession: '. . . and I went to the doctor with my cough and he never examined my chest, never even looked up but just wrote me out a prescription and so I've come here doctor'. If a patient walks into the A&E consulting room complaining of an ankle injury, a normal gait makes the presence of a fracture highly unlikely. The ankle still needs to be fully examined for the reasons stated above but the absence of a fracture could be confirmed by localizing the tenderness to the lateral ligament of the ankle rather than the bone (see Chapter 30), an examination which will take a few seconds only. However, if the patient is unhappy, any explanations about why an X-ray is unnecessary and how to treat a minor sprain will be more time-consuming. A full examination may therefore not just leave the patient more satisfied but may save time in the long run. Clearly time should not be wasted on a pointless examination but to to do slightly more than is strictly necessary may be appropriate.

It is worth recording one's *uncritical* impressions of patients. If the patient is unduly anxious, tearful, or aggressive, the fact should be noted but it should not be forgotten that patients are entitled to see their medical records and comments must be fair and supportable. There is no place for being rude about patients in the notes whether this is written in plain language or described in coded form or abbreviation.

It has been noted above that many patients sustain their injuries while under the influence of alcohol. If a patient smells of alcohol, it should be noted but many diseases can mimic intoxication. The word 'drunk' is best avoided and a diagnosis of alcohol intoxication should never be made without a full physical examination being recorded in the notes and preferably a history of alcohol intake which supports the diagnosis. It is too easy to dismiss the head-injured patient who has consumed one drink as drunk because he smells of alcohol and is acting strangely and thereby miss a treatable condition. Measuring the blood alcohol does not solve the problem as the relationship between the blood alcohol level and conscious level is very variable. Also even proving that the patient is intoxicated does not exclude an associated significant injury (but possibly makes it more likely). A medical problem which may not only be confused with alcohol intoxication but which can also be caused by it, is hypoglycaemia. Every patient who smells of alcohol and who has a diminished level of consciousness must have their blood sugar recorded.

To support (and therefore to make) a diagnosis of alcohol intoxication the A&E records should contain notes such as:

'*History*:
Found by ambulance crew outside pub
Was able to stagger into ambulance

Vomited × 1 in ambulance
Friends say he has consumed at least 10 pints beer and
2 double whiskies
Denies any injury.
PMH: ? — can't give details.
O/E: Smells of alcohol + + +. Flushed, no cyanosis or jaundice.
No external evidence of trauma.
CVS:
P100 SR, BP 115/80
Ht Sounds I&II NAD
RS: Chest clear.
Abdo:
Soft, no tenderness, scars, masses
Liver, spleen, kidneys not felt
Bowel sound NAD.
CNS:
GCS E 3
       V 4 (telling me to f*** off)
       M 6
Pupils dilated but same size and both react to light
Nystagmus to left and right gaze
Power left = right
Reflexes Left = right = present but reduced plantars
Blood sugar: 6 mmol/l
Diagnosis: Alcohol intoxication'

In the absence of supporting evidence in the form of a knowledge of intake and a negative general examination the diagnosis would have to remain 'Confusional state in association
with alcohol intake' until intoxication could be proved either
by measuring the blood alcohol or by the passage of time (i.e.
the patient gets better spontaneously over a few hours).

An episode of intoxication which results in an injury may
be an isolated occurrence but the possibility of alcoholism
should be considered. A suitable, brief screening test which
can be applied in the A&E department is the CAGE questionnaire.[1] This consists of four non-incriminating questions:

1. 'Have you ever felt that you should **C**ut down on your
drinking?'
2. 'Have people **A**nnoyed you by criticizing your drinking?'

3. 'Have you ever felt bad or **G**uilty about your drinking?'
4. 'Have you ever had a drink first thing in the morning to steady your nerves or to get rid of a hangover (**E**ye-opener)?'

Positive responses to two or more questions is a sensitive indicator for alcoholism.

How much information to record

Notes on a neurological examination which would satisfy a professor of neurology on his ward round might fill two sides of A4 paper. This would be unnecessary and inappropriate for most A&E patients. Even more inappropriate for a head-injured patient is an examination note which reads:

'CNS—NAD'

as this does not indicate what examination has been done. However, there are occasions in A&E when both might be appropriate. A two-page neurological examination may be needed in a patient with some abnormal neurological signs or who has unusual symptoms following a head injury. The examination note 'CNS—NAD' will never be adequate for anyone who has suffered a head or spinal injury but may be appropriate if a patient has fallen and sustained injuries of both ankles and a wrist. In these circumstances one needs to exclude any other injury and one may write:

'No evidence of injury to head, neck, spine, chest, abdomen, pelvis, CNS—NAD . . .' (see Chapter 37).

If one does write this, one must be able to say what examination was actually done, does it mean 'appeared alert (but I didn't formally test whether he was orientated) and moving all four limbs' or were pupils looked at, reflexes tapped etc.

Reference

1. Mayfield, D., McLeod, G., & Hall, P. (1974). The CAGE questionnaire: validation of a new alcoholism screening instrument. *American Journal of Psychiatry*, **131**, 1121–3.

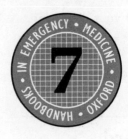

CHAPTER 7

Provisional or differential diagnosis

It is important that this is written down as only by formally comparing the final diagnosis reached after X-rays or other investigations with this provisional diagnosis will clinical diagnostic skills improve. Following an ankle injury the provisional diagnosis could read:

'Probably a sprain, but X-ray as won't weight bear'

or

'Possible fracture lateral malleollus'

It is also important as a means of avoiding diagnostic errors because if the provisional diagnosis reads: 'Clinical bimalleolar fracture', and the ankle X-ray is normal, one should think again and possibly request additional X-ray views or ask advice. This is particularly relevant when one doctor requests an X-ray and then goes off duty leaving somebody else to look at the films.

Every **X-ray** or other **investigation** requested should be listed. (If the A&E department is computerized, tick the appropriate boxes on the casualty card as well.) If a patient has hip, knee, and ankle injuries it is not enough to write 'XR—NBI' as this gives no indication as to which of the three has been X-rayed. When requesting an X-ray be very careful about stating the side of the injury and if you use sticky labels, ensure that you have stuck the correct label on the request form. The X-ray request form is a request for a radiologist's opinion and the X-ray report will be more accu-

24

rate and useful if the radiologist is in full possession of the facts. He or she needs to know the type of injury suspected but also about previous fractures or other medical problems which may be relevant. The X-ray request should not read 'ankle injury—X-ray ankle please' but:

'Inversion injury, tender lateral malleollus, NB previous Ca breast—X-ray ankle please'

Another reason for stating the injury you wish to exclude on the X-ray request form is that it enables the radiographer to do appropriate X-rays. For example, the exposures required to show glass foreign bodies will be different from those used to show a fracture and a fractured calcaneum is shown much better on calcaneal views than on an ankle X-ray. If an X-ray request states '? fracture calcaneum—X-ray ankle' the radiographer should do calcaneum views even though these have not been specifically requested. This advantage will not be gained by the 'ankle injury—please X-ray' type of request.

The doctor's interpretation of every investigation should be recorded. The interpretation of an X-ray should not just state whether or not the suspected fracture is present but should be the equivalent of a radiologist's report. If a chest X-ray taken for trauma shows a carcinoma of the lung as an incidental finding, a note which says 'CXR—NBI' may be true but unhelpful. Even clinically insignificant abnormalities should be noted because unless they are first seen it is impossible to decide on their significance. It also makes the job more interesting and less of a production line if every now and again for example the changes of a long-standing primary tuberculosis or of some minor congenital variation in anatomy are seen. Where X-ray findings are equivocal their interpretation may depend on re-examining the patient. This should be reflected in the records e.g. an ankle X-ray may be described as:

'Curious appearance of medial malleollus but not tender there so not a fracture'.

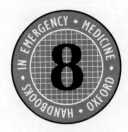

CHAPTER 8

Final diagnosis

Diagnosis is fundamental to medicine. The diagnosis you make will label the patient. It may be entered into a computer, copied into the general practitioner's notes, and will be referred to in the absence of the rest of the clinical notes. It may be coded and used to generate statistics. It is therefore important that the diagnosis is as complete as possible. 'Fall' or 'injury right hand' are not diagnoses. 'Fractured right 4th metacarpal' is a diagnosis but better still is 'Undisplaced transverse fracture base right 4th metacarpal'.

It is important to describe fully a fracture, not just for the notes but also so that it can be described to someone else, for example if one needs to ask advice on further management. When describing a fracture the following should be noted:

- Closed or compound (if compound, the wound needs to be described as well).
- Location, e.g. for a long bone: base, midshaft, junction of upper ⅓ and lower ⅔.
- Type e.g. transverse, oblique, spiral, comminuted, segmental, greenstick, epiphyseal (what type?).
- Displacement i.e. undisplaced or displaced.
- The type of displacement e.g. shift, angulation, rotation.

Two very different fractures of the tibia could be described:

'Undisplaced transverse fracture midshaft tibia with intact fibula'

or

'Compound oblique fracture lower ⅓ tibia with 15° anterior angulation of lower fragment associated with fracture of midshaft fibula'

26

A complete diagnosis must be accurate and must be supported by the clinical findings. All too often soft tissue knee problems are diagnosed as '? meniscus injury' or even 'meniscus injury', when it is clear from the notes that the real diagnosis is a sprain or a contusion. If one is unable to make a definite diagnosis one should give the most accurate diagnosis it is possible to make at the time e.g. 'STI left knee, ? medial collateral ligament sprain, ? medial meniscus' or if one is less certain, 'STI left knee ? exact nature'. This allows the diagnosis to be refined at a later date and avoids the patient being mislabelled and so mismanaged.

The final diagnosis must also take into consideration not just the injury but also any medical problem which caused the injury. For example, the fact that a patient had a cardiac arrhythmia and fell is probably much more important than their undisplaced Colles' fracture.

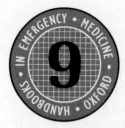

CHAPTER 9

Treatment

Drugs

The A&E record card may be used for prescribing drugs given in the department. Any prescription made in this way must contain the same information as any other prescription.

Drug dosage, frequency, and duration (or total number of tablets prescribed) should be written down even if the prescribing is being done on a separate form. It is not helpful when a patient returns and requests more medication to find that all that is written in the notes is 'ibuprofen' without any mention of dose and frequency of administration or, even worse, 'NSAIDs'.

Drug doses (especially in children) are frequently given in milligrams per kilogram. It is often not possible to weigh an ill child and so approximations need to be used. It is important that calculations are written down and it is usually most appropriate if these and any assumptions made are written in the notes, e.g.

'Mother says 3 stone = (approx) 18 kg
Pethidine 1–2 mg/kg
so 20 mg pethidine IM stat'

or

'Age = 3, mean weight = 2(age + 4) so weight = approx 14 kg—say 15 kg
Normal saline 20 ml/kg so 300 ml'

or

'Weight = 55 kg
N acetyl cysteine 150 mg/kg in 15 mins
so 8.25 g'

For complicated calculations and toxic drugs, it is important that any arithmetic and the position of the decimal point is checked (preferably by someone else who should also sign the card).

Before giving any drug, ask about past medical history, other medication, and allergies. If a patient claims to be allergic to a drug one should ask (and note) what form the allergy took. Diarrhoea following antibiotics may falsely be regarded by the patient as an allergy and it is clearly important to differentiate between the penicillin allergy that caused a rash and that which caused anaphylaxis. Similarly any warnings given to patients about drugs should also be noted. Examples of appropriate notes are:

'PMH—nil significant, drugs—nil, allergies—nil ibuprofen 400 mg qds 7/7'
'Penicillin V 250 mg qds (not allergic)'

'PMH mild indigestion, no proven ulcer. No allergies. Ibuprofen 400 mg qds (with food), stop if indigestion worsens'

or

'Allergic to penicillin—generalized rash—for erythromycin 500 mg qds 7/7'

Practical procedures

Many types of practical procedure are performed in A&E departments either for treatment or investigation. These should be described in the same detail as would be done if the same procedure was being performed in an operating theatre. The type of anaesthesia should be noted as should the position of any incisions. Tourniquet time should be recorded.

Wound repair is more than just suturing. The opportunity

provided by the local anaesthesia required for this should be taken to fully clean and debride the wound and to explore its depths to exclude other injury. These should all be described e.g.:

'1% lignocaine digital nerve block
wound cleaned and scrubbed, ragged bits of skin trimmed, explored, small (< 20%) laceration in extensor tendon. Tendon left. 5 × 4/0 ethilon to skin'

Recording the number of sutures will help the person who has to remove them.

After manipulation describe the method of anaesthesia, the name of the anaesthetist, the method of reduction (where appropriate), and give some indication of the ease of reduction, the stability of the reduction etc. If there are known complications of the injury or its treatment, record that you looked for them. For example, for a dislocated shoulder:

'Diazepam 15 mg IV and entonox
Easy reduction (Kocher's method)
Sling
Post-reduction X-ray—confirms reduction
Axillary nerve—sensation intact'

or, for a fracture of the distal radius:

'MUA fracture distal third radius Dr...... GA Dr.......
Difficult reduction, very unstable
Long arm POP wrist flexed neutral rotation
Post-reduction X-ray—good position
Sling
Will need a further X-ray next week'

There is only one way to document the position of a fracture after manipulation or to confirm that a dislocation has been reduced and that is by a post reduction X-ray which must be requested in every case.

Joint aspiration

Record the site of aspiration, the volume, and nature of aspirate and whether it has been sent for microbiological investigation. The patient is usually much more comfortable after a large effusion has been drained from a joint and so the opportunity should be taken to re-examine the joint and record the findings. For example, in a patient with a large knee effusion in whom it was difficult to exclude instability because of pain the note of the aspiration might read:

'Aspiration Right knee Dr......
Cleaned with iodine   1% lignocaine
Medial approach
70 ml heavily blood-stained fluid aspirated
After aspiration pain much easier. On re-examination:
ROM now 10–130°, stable . . .'

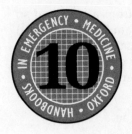

CHAPTER 10

Advice to patients and follow-up

A summary of the advice given to patients including any printed information given and any referral should be noted. For a sprained ankle it would not be too much to note:

'Crepe bandage
crutches
advised ice, elevation, keep moving
referred physiotherapy
advice sheet given
has paracetamol at home'

Sometimes there are several possible treatments and the options are discussed with the patient. For example for a finger tip injury the notes might read:

'Pros and cons of conservative v. operative treatment discussed. For terminalization'

A patient's refusal of treatment should be noted and where this might have serious consequences, the refusal should be confirmed by the patient's signature on the appropriate form. If they refuse even to sign the form, this must be confirmed by the signature of a witness on the records.

Follow-up

The discharge of the patient should be noted as should any instructions the patient is given about what to do should their problem get worse or fail to improve e.g.:

'See A&E clinic 5/7. Return earlier if more pain or if becomes pyrexial'

or

'Discharged, see GP if no better in 2 weeks'.

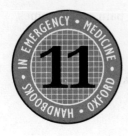

CHAPTER 11

Letters to the general practitioner

Key points in letters to the GP
- Consider what information the GP needs to know.

General practitioners have the responsibility for the continuing care of the patient and so should be informed of their patient's attendance at the A&E department. Many A&E departments will send a computer-generated letter to the GP and most will have proforma letters which can be filled in. For the vast majority of attendances information can be communicated by a letter such as:

Dear Dr ....

The above named patient attended this department today.

Diagnosis: Laceration scalp, left parietal region
X-ray: Skull XR—NBI
Treatment: Sutured under LA, 8 sutures
               Tetanus toxoid booster
Follow-up: Please remove sutures in 1 week

Yours sincerely,

However, it is important to consider what information the GP needs to manage the patient. He or she needs to follow-up the wound, and the above information is adequate for that but on occasions the reason for the accident is even more important. It may be more important for the GP to know that the laceration was caused by being assaulted by a spouse or was caused by being intoxicated at 10 a.m. than to be told that there is a wound (which will be obvious). Complex medical and social problems cannot be communicated by means of a simple proforma and so require a letter. A carbon copy (or photocopy) of the a letter should be kept in the notes. Usually the patient will be asked to deliver the letter to the GP themselves but in some cases, it may be more appropriate to send it in the post.

PART 2

Musculoskeletal injuries and wounds

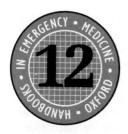

CHAPTER 12

Joint injuries

The examination of a joint can be summarized as:

- Look (inspection).
- Feel (palpation).
- Move.
- Special tests.
- Function.

In doing this one should always compare the injured side with the uninjured side.

Look

The joint should be inspected for:

- Position in which the joint is held.
- Deformity.
- Wounds, bruising, redness.
- Old scars, sinuses etc. (indicating previous injuries or pathology).
- Swelling or effusion.
- Muscle wasting (indicating long-standing problems).

Feel

The most important thing to feel for is to identify the point of maximum tenderness. For example in the ankle, if the

39

most tender point is over a malleollus then a fracture is a possibility but if the maximum tenderness is over the soft tissues then a significant fracture is unlikely.

The presence of an effusion may be easier to feel than to see. It is important to differentiate between an effusion and other causes of swelling, such as haematoma, oedema, fluid in a bursa, or a long-standing problem such as synovial thickening. This can usually be determined by palpation. Deformity may also frequently be more easily felt than seen.

Move

The normal range of movement in a joint is very variable though some 'averages' are described in each chapter. For an individual the normal range of movement in a joint can best be determined by comparison with the uninjured side. When this is not possible, either because the uninjured joint has pre-existing disease or, in the spine where there is no uninjured side to compare, a normal range can only be estimated by experience of patients of similar age and build.

Clearly, moving a joint will be omitted (or at least postponed until after the reassurance of a normal X-ray) if inspection and palpation suggest a strong possibility of a significant injury. One should examine first the active and then the passive range of movement (ROM) and this should be recorded using the convention that the fully extended anatomical position of an extremity is 0°.[1] Thus the normal range of movement of the elbow is 0–150° (not 180–30°). If movements are reduced, notes saying 'Decreased ROM' means very little. The reduction in movement is measurable and should be recorded e.g. 'ROM 30–90°'. This gives a measure against which improvement or deterioration can be judged. Alternatively one can write: 'full flexion, lacks 20° extension', 'full range of movement except for the last 10° of flexion' or, for a longstanding problem 'fixed flexion deformity of 15°, full flexion'. If the range of movement of a joint is reduced it can be assumed that this is because of pain but if the patient has full movement, the presence of pain should be noted e.g. 'full ROM but pain at extremes' or 'full ROM but pain on flexing beyond 90°'. The presence of crepitus should also be noted.

The stability of a joint should be examined under the heading of movement and any ligamentous laxity compared to the uninjured side.

Special tests

The history and examination should suggest a differential diagnosis which may need special tests to clarify e.g. if rupture of the extensor mechanism of the knee needs to be excluded, the ability to straight leg raise or extend the knee against gravity will need to be assessed.

Function

The examination of a joint should include an examination of its function. The principal function of the lower limbs is walking and it is essential therefore to examine the gait (unless the patient clearly has an injury which contra-indicates this). Even if the physical examination of the supine patient is unremarkable an inability to weight bear or to walk only with difficulty should raise the suspicion of a significant injury and suggest a need to re-examine the patient or to radiographs. Many a patient had injuries missed simply because they were not asked to walk. A normal gait will exclude many injuries (see also Chapter 27).

Lastly, the examination of any joint should include an examination of the joint above and below. Pain may be referred (e.g. hip pain being felt in the knee) and, especially in small children and others unable to give an accurate history, it is not uncommon to localize incorrectly the site of injury (e.g. for the patient to present as an ankle injury but for there to be a fracture in the foot). It is also not rare for a patient to have two injuries in a limb e.g. a fall on the outstretched hand causing both a Colles' fracture and a fracture of the radial head.

Note keeping for a joint injury

The notes of the examination of a joint injury should, as a minimum, *always* include details of:

- Presence or absence of any effusion or swelling.
- Point of maximum tenderness.
- Range of movement.
- Stability.
- Gait (lower limb injuries).

However, much more detail may need to be included. Examples of note keeping are given later in chapters devoted to specific joints.

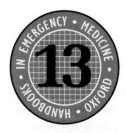

CHAPTER 13

Bone injuries

The examination of a bone can be summarized as:

- Look.
- Feel.
- Move.
- Special tests.
- Examine the joint at each end.

Look

As with a joint injury, a bone should be inspected for:

- Position in which the limb is held.
- Deformity.
- Wounds, bruising, redness.
- Old scars, sinuses etc. (indicating previous injuries or pathology).
- Swelling.
- Muscle wasting (indicating long-standing problems).
- The joint at each end should be inspected.

Feel

The following can be felt:

- Point of maximum tenderness.
- Any deformity may be more easily felt than seen.
- Any swelling can be localized.
- The temperature compared to the other side.

Move

If there is an obvious fracture the limb should not be moved unnecessarily but it may be necessary, even if just to splint the limb. If the limb is moved then the presence of crepitus should be noted. In less severe injuries, the limb will be moved as part of the examination of the joints at either end. If there is doubt as to whether there is a fracture or whether a known fracture has healed, then the bone can be stressed.

Special tests

If there is an obvious fracture, the circulation and nerve supply to the limb distal to the fracture should always be examined. Commonly associated injuries should be looked for.

Notekeeping for a bony injury

The following should *always* be noted:

- Presence or absence of deformity and swelling.
- Point of maximum tenderness.
- Examination of the joint at each end.
- Function.

If there is a fracture with deformity, the condition of the skin overlying the fracture should be commented on and the vascular and nerve supply distally should be recorded (see Chapters 34 and 35). The notes of the examination of a fracture might read:

'Obviously displaced Pott's fracture, skin stretched tight over bony prominence of medial malleollus and blanched. Foot warm, pulses present, good capillary return. Sensation in foot intact.'

The above injury needs to be reduced as soon as possible to improve the blood supply to the skin through which a surgeon is shortly going to want to cut and also to avoid the stretching of the blood vessels and nerves which cross the fracture. If this is done immediately before the limb is X-rayed, there will be no record of the severity of the injury when it was first seen. Such a record can be made with a photograph which should become part of the notes.

If the fracture is compound, the wound itself should be fully described and tendon and nerve injury should be excluded (see below).

Once it has been inspected, the wound overlying a compound fracture should be dressed and left undisturbed until surgery. A Polaroid photograph of the wound facilitates this and allows the surgeon to know what the wound looks like. Instant photographs should be immediately marked with the patient's name and the date lest they get separated from the rest of the clinical records.

Examples of notes on fractures are given later in chapters relating to specific injuries.

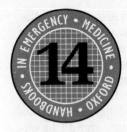

CHAPTER 14

Wounds

Key points in wounds

- A diagram is worth a thousand words.
- Test tendon and nerve function distal to every wound.

History

As noted above (p. 14) the mechanism of the wounding may give valuable clues as to the type of injuries sustained. Other questions one may need to ask include the direction of a penetrating injury, the length of a blade causing a stab wound (NB the length of the track may be longer than the length of the blade due to the elasticity of the tissues), and whether there is the possibility of a foreign body (especially with thorn injuries—ask 'did the point of the thorn come out?'). The time the wound occurred is important when considering whether to primarily close it and for deciding on tetanus prophylaxis.

All patients with wounds should be asked about their tetanus immunization status. This falls into into three groups:

1. Patient has had a full course of tetanus toxoid injections or a booster following a full course within the previous 10 years.

2. The patient has had a full course of tetanus toxoid injections or a booster following a full course more than 10 years ago.

3. The patient has never had a full course of tetanus toxoid injections or the tetanus status is unknown.

It is not sufficient to write in the notes 'tetanus injection 5 years ago' and to assume that the patient is protected. Ensure that the patient has had a full course by asking about normal childhood injections (many patients do not realize that the triple vaccine includes tetanus toxoid) and military service (patients who have served in the military can be assumed to have had a course of tetanus toxoid at that time). If a patient says they are allergic to tetanus toxoid, ask further questions about the reaction. A local reaction is not an allergic response and does not contraindicate further injections. A severe generalized allergic response is likely to have been due to horse serum which is no longer used.

Examination

The following should be noted:

- Type of wound.
- Location.
- Direction and shape.
- Size (length and width).
- Depth.
- Evidence of underlying bony injury.
- Nerve and tendon function distal to the wound.

Type of wound

There is an obvious difference between a gunshot wound and a laceration but differentiate also between a cleanly incised wound and the more ragged and bruised appearance of a wound caused by a blunt force. Is the wound clean or dirty?—tidy or untidy?—is there skin loss?

Location, direction, and shape

The location of the wound should be described as accurately as possible and the direction should be described as transverse, longitudinal or oblique. The shape should be described (e.g. Y-shaped, stellate). If the wound is a flap, it should be noted whether it is proximally or distally based. The viability of the flap should be commented on. This information is frequently best shown on a diagram or drawing and most A&E departments have rubber stamps of different parts of the body for the less artistic to use.

Size

The size of the wound, haematoma, flap, skin loss, etc. should be stated. Sometimes this will need exact measurement but usually an approximation will be sufficient. Similarly, if a wound infection is present one should measure the extent of the erythema to give a baseline against which improvement or deterioration can be measured. An additional means of establishing such a baseline is to draw round the edge of the erythema with a pen. When the patient is seen later for review, it is obvious, without measurement, whether the extent of the redness is greater or less.

The measurement of a wound need not necessarily be in centimetres but can be described in relation to the anatomy. For example, 'longditudinal laceration on dorsum of finger from PIP joint to DIP joint' or 'transverse laceration lower shin, junction of middle and lower third, about half the circumference'.

Partial thickness skin loss will usually heal well and so for abrasions or for areas of skin loss it is often more important to know the area of the full thickness loss. For example, 'abrasion 5 × 4 cm, mostly superficial but small area 1 cm^2 full thickness loss of skin in centre'.

The location, size, and shape of wounds can also be documented by a photograph. Clearly, not every wound should be photographed but if there is a reason (e.g. for teaching, for accident prevention purposes, to document a complex wound or for medicolegal reasons) take a photograph and label it with the date and patient's name.

When determining the rate of healing of ulcers or other wounds (e.g. for clinical trials), an accurate measurement of the area can be made by tracing round the edge of the ulcer on to a piece of tracing paper and measuring the area from a grid. The tracing of the wound forms part of the records and can be used for future comparisons. This is not needed for the acute management of patients at their first attendace at A&E.

Depth

Some indication should be given of the depth of the wound. Mention of the depth of abrasions and skin loss has been made above but the same should be done with lacerations. Depth can be indicated in such ways as 'very superficial', 'through skin alone', 'through skin, superficial fascia and into muscle' or 'wound through to skull, periosteum intact'. The depth of the wound may be further clarified when it is explored as part of its cleaning and suturing. Exclusion of tendon or nerve injury is done, not by peering into a wound, but by the examination of function distal to it (see below). If there is any possibility of a radiopaque foreign body, the wound should be X-rayed. If on inspecting a wound one observes a tendon end, arterial bleeding, a divided nerve or foreign material, this should be recorded.

Evidence of a bony injury

Wounds caused by a blunt force may harbour a fracture of the underlying bone. Fractures of the tibia will not easily be overlooked as the patient is not weight-bearing, however, elsewhere (e.g. the 'nightstick' fracture of the midshaft of the ulna) compound fractures may be overlooked if one concentrates on the wound alone. In all wounds, evidence of a fracture should be investigated. The detection of bony tenderness may be difficult to determine but joint movements and function should be recorded.

Evidence of tendon and nerve injury

Tendon and nerve injuries are frequently missed. It is essential that tendon and nerve function are tested distal to every limb wound, no matter how superficial it seems. Wounds may be deeper than they appear and nerves (especially the median nerve at the wrist and the digital nerves), may be very superficial. Those tendons and nerves tested will depend on the location of the wound but it should not be forgotten that a penetrating wound may divide a structure a long way from the entry point. The examination of a nerve injury is described in Chapter 35.

When missed tendon injuries are finally diagnosed, the previous notes will be referred to and will often contain vague statements such as 'tendons and nerves intact'.[1] This calls into question what examination was done to support the statement and this must be made clear in the notes. The examination of normal tendon and nerve function distal to a laceration of the anterior wrist should read as a minimum:

'FDP √√√√ FDS √√√√ FCU √ FCR √ FPL √
Ulna n √   Median n √   ,

However, the examination of the nerves could be even better recorded as described in Chapter 35.

Reference

1. Guly, H. R. (1991). Missed tendon injuries. *Archives of Emergency Medicine*, **8**, 87–91.

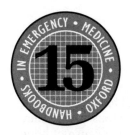

CHAPTER 15

Non-traumatic problems

Patients with acute musculoskeletal pains commonly presented to the A&E department as do patients with less acute problems. It is not the function of this book to give advice on whether these patients should be seen or treated in an emergency department but if they are seen (even if referred back to their general practitioner for treatment) it is important that their problems are assessed and documented properly.

History

As with traumatic problems it is of vital importance to try to establish the exact sequence of events. The first question is to establish is 'When did the problem first start?' or 'When were you last completely well?' and the second question is 'What was the first thing you noticed wrong?' It is also important to try to discover what the patient was doing during the time leading up to the start of the symptoms as many musculoskeletal pains have their origin in overuse (e.g. in sport, at work or with unaccustomed do-it-yourself activities). Not infrequently, seemingly non-traumatic problems do, in fact, have their origin in an injury. From this description of the the start of the problem one can establish the progression or alteration in symptoms and the response to any treatment. Patients with musculoskeletal problems may have sought help from an osteopath or chiropracter as well as from a doctor. This may not be volunteered and so may need to be asked about. Most patients present with pain. Ask about:

● Exact location of pain.
● Nature of pain.

- Any change in severity or nature.
- Radiation of pain.
- Factors which ease the pain.
- Factors which worsen the pain.
- Response to treatment.

In non-traumatic problems the past medical history is of even more importance than it is for injuries. Previous malignancy will suggest the possibility of metastases as a cause of bone pain or a history of iritis in a patient presenting with an acutely painful knee may indicate Reiter's syndrome and should prompt enquiry about diarrhoea and urethritis.

It is important to establish what effect a patient's problem has on their life and activities and so a knowledge of their occupation and recreational interests is vital. This may also, on occasion, help with establishing a diagnosis. As with traumatic problems it is important to use the history taking as a means of establishing a relationship with the patient and trying to understand why the patient has sought help. If a patient attends 'inappropriately' it is important to ask why they have come to A&E rather than to their general practitioner and if they have a chronic problem one needs to discover what precipitated their decision to attend. A brief family history will often need to be taken and this may be as simple and brief as:

'Does anybody else in the family have joint problems?'

Not only are there some diseases which run in families but a family history may alert one to any hidden fears such as a fear of malignancy. A parent who has lost a child with leukaemia will worry considerably that any ache or pain in another child is the same problem. If at all possible such information must be discovered so that reassurance can be given (and if necessary), further investigations done. Any such hidden fears discovered should be recorded to help any other doctor who treats the patient.

Examination

As with the examination of patients following a musculoskeletal injury the examination should follow the following pattern:

- Look.
- Feel.
- Move.
- Function.
- Special tests.

Non-traumatic joint pain

History

Arthritic pain is common and the causes are numerous but in A&E practice other causes of joint pain (e.g. bursitis, un-recognized injury, tendinitis, referred pain) are probably commoner than arthritis in its various types. So numerous are the possible causes of pain in a joint that it is not always easy to make a diagnosis. It should go without saying that it is necessary to take a full history, past history (especially of joint problems), and family history as previously described. In addition, in appropriate cases, it may be necessary to ask specific questions if the answers have not been obtained by more open questioning and to note the answers. Examples of such direct questions concern:

- Morning stiffness (suggests an inflammatory arthritis).
- History of gout.
- History of bleeding disorders.
- History of recent viral illness (common as a cause of an arthritis in children).
- History of conjunctivitis, iritis, urethritis, diarrhoea (may suggest Reiter's disease).
- History of trauma.

Non-traumatic bone pain

History

If a patient points at a bone as the site of their pain, it is important, first, to establish whether the pain does have its origin in the bone or whether it is from some other structure such as a muscle insertion. Typically, bone pain is described as a boring pain, worse at night and pain from muscles and tendons will be worse on exertion. Pain from a stress fracture will also be exacerbated by exercise. Some of the commoner causes of bone pain are:

- Osteomyelitis.
- Tumours (metastases are more common than primary tumours).
- Stress fracture.
- Paget's disease (possibly with a stress fracture).
- Unrecognized trauma (especially in small children).

and the ways in which these present are varied but ask about:

- Past medical history:
  –general,
  –previous problems in the specific area.
- Trauma
- Systemic symptoms (e.g. pyrexia, loss of appetite, others).
- Recent heavy exertion.

Negative as well as positive responses should be noted.

Examination

The examination of a patient with pain in the region of a bone should differentiate between true bone pain and referred pain or pain from other nearby or attached structures. This will involve the same type of examination as described above for patients with bony injuries. However, when there is any possibility of the pain being due to an osteomyelitis, it is essential that the patient's temperature is taken and the presence or absence of local inflammation (redness, warmth etc.) be recorded.

Example of note keeping

History:
Last week, fell and injured lower leg, bruised shin but no limping, no wound, continued to play normally

Yesterday complained of pain in leg, limped
Last night pain kept him awake, not helped by paracetamol.
This a.m., pain ++, won't weight bear.
DQ:
Well in self until this a.m., had normal tea yesterday
Didn't eat this a.m.
No diarrhoea, vomiting, no other pains.
PMH: Nil significant.
Drugs: Nil.
O/E:
Acutely tender upper tibia at junction upper ¼ and lower ¾
Slight redness and oedema
No inguinal modes
Pyrexial—T 38.4 °C (axilla)
No abnormality of knee or ankle, full ROM.
Diagnosis: probable osteomyelitis.

Examination

The examination of the uninjured but painful joint is the
same as for an injured joint but the emphasis is different.
Muscle wasting is more likely to be obvious in a longer
standing problem than following an acute injury. Many
causes of joint pain including arthritis, bursitis and overlying soft tissue sepsis will have an inflammatory cause and
signs of inflammation must always be looked for and their
presence (or absence) recorded.

Not only must the active and passive ranges of movement
be examined as described above, but if the pain might be
caused by a tendonitis, the power of the muscles whose
tendons traverse the joint must be examined (resisted movements). For example, if resisted shoulder abduction causes
pain in the absence of any movement at the shoulder joint,
the provoked pain must have its origin in the supraspinatus
muscle or tendon.

Referred pain is probably more common in non-traumatic
problems and therefore the joints above and below should
be examined, especially if no abnormality is found on examining the painful joint.

A general examination is often necessary and particularly
if a septic condition has entered the differential diagnosis,

the notes are not complete without a record of the patient's temperature, and the possibility of gout should prompt a search for tophi.

Inexplicable symptoms

On occasion a patient may present with either very vague symptoms in a limb or with other symptoms which the doctor finds totally inexplicable despite a full history and initial examination. This should lead to the search being wide for a cause of the symptoms. For example, pain in the upper limb may be caused by diseases of the: musculoskeletal system, nerves (spinal cord, nerve roots, brachial plexus, peripheral nerves, reflex sympathetic dystrophy), or blood vessels and some types of pain may be referred from the heart, pleura, or diaphragm. Thus, for a patient with unexplained upper limb pain direct questions may need to be asked about chest and cardiac symptoms and if these are negative an examination might be recorded as:

'Neck: not tender, full ROM. Movements do not reproduce pain
No tenderness whole upper limb from finger tips to SC joint
Full painless ROM shoulder, elbow, radioulnar, wrist, fingers
Power L = R = strong in all muscle groups. All painless
Sensation to light touch L = R = normal, no hyperaesthesia
Reflexes:

	Right	Left
BJ	++	++
TJ	++	++
SJ	++	++

Pulses all present, L = R, no bruits
Temperature of skin L = R
Symptoms not reproduced by downward pull on arms
P 86, BP 130/85, normal heart sounds
Chest clear
Diagnosis: ?'

If the patient volunteers that musculoskeletal symptoms are worse after exercise, send him or her for a walk round the hospital grounds (or whatever other exercise is likely to worsen the symptoms) and re-examine him or her.

In other circumstances the possibility of a non-organic cause may be considered. A psychological cause for symptoms must never be diagnosed solely on the absence of an obvious physical cause but must be supported in the notes by positive features of psychiatric or psychological illness. Questions can be asked about psychiatric and social problems and the patient's own attitude to the symptoms. However, in A&E where one is unlikely to have previous knowledge of the patient it should be normally be assumed that symptoms have an organic basis unless there is very good evidence to the contrary (the presence of psychological problems does not exclude associated physical disease). Doctors must accept they do not know everything.

Soft tissue infections

Soft tissue infections have traditionally been seen and treated in A&E departments. On occasion it may be difficult to differentiate between a cellulitis and the presence of an abscess. In such patients, throbbing pain which kept them awake the previous night is highly suggestive of pus under pressure and is almost always an indication for incision. Apart from a proper description of the position and extent of the infection the following should be noted:

History:
• Did the pain keep them awake last night? (see above).
• Trauma.
• Previous infections.
• Systemic symptoms (e.g. pyrexia).
• Response to antibiotics (if given).

Examination:
• Temperature.
• Presence of enlarged draining lymph nodes.

PART 3

Parts of the body

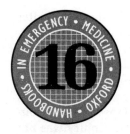

CHAPTER 16

Head injury

History

It is important to ask enough questions to understand fully the mechanism of the head injury. A fall on to concrete is more likely to cause a fracture than a fall on to a carpeted floor. A high velocity deceleration injury such as a road accident is likely to cause severe generalized neuronal injury whereas a blow by a hard object may fracture the skull but cause little brain injury. If the object causing the blow is small, such as a hammer, the patient may have a compound depressed fracture, the severity of which may not be appreciated if the patient never lost consciousness. A penetrating injury such as an an attack with a screwdriver is unlikely to cause a loss of consciousness but will also put the patient at risk of intracranial infection if not diagnosed and properly treated.

The mechanism of injury is also important for appreciating the possibility of associated injuries. A moving head which strikes a stationary object is likely to cause a cervical spine injury as well as the presenting head injury whereas this is not likely to occur if a moving object hits a stationary head.

It is important also to ask about the sequence of events. Did the patient lose consciousness and then fall, striking their head, or did they trip, hit their head, and become unconscious as a result of the head injury? In the patient who has had a head injury and who had a fit it is important to try to determine whether the fit caused the head injury or was a complication of the head injury.

One must also ask how the patient was immediately after the injury. This question must be asked of people who witnessed the event, who will describe the patient's state in words, and of the first ambulance personnel at the scene who should also be able to describe the conscious level using the Glasgow Coma Score (GCS). If a patient was fully conscious immediately after the accident and then lapsed into unconsciousness, it is clear that the primary brain injury was not severe and that the cause of the coma is a secondary insult which may be treatable. Many an extradural haematoma has been missed because a patient brought into hospital unconscious was assumed to have been in that state since the accident. If a patient's level of consciousness has fallen since they were first seen it is important to enquire how this happened. A sudden loss of consciousness suggests that the patient may have had a fit even if this was not witnessed but a gradual loss of consciousness might suggest other causes such as shock, hypoxia or intracranial haematoma. On the other hand, if the patient had a GCS of 10 when first seen but on arrival at hospital the GCS has risen to 14, this is clearly a good sign. A pupil which was fixed and dilated when the ambulance arrived a few minutes after the accident is likely to represent local trauma but a pupil which was normal and dilated later is more serious. In addition to asking whether the patient lost consciousness, it is also important to note the duration of post-traumatic amnesia. This is a measure of head injury severity and an indicator of the prognosis. Post-traumatic amnesia is defined as the time until continuing memory returns. This is determined by asking: 'What is the next thing you remember after the accident?' This question should be repeated before discharge.

The past medical history of a patient with a head injury is of vital importance. Pre-existing neurological abnormalities may wrongly be assumed to be due to the head injury as may pupillary abnormalities due to ophthalmic disease or eye drops. Similarly one must also be careful not to attribute all neurological signs to pre-existing disease unless there is good evidence for this. Anticoagulant therapy may predispose to intracranial haematoma as may treated hydrocephalus or brain atrophy (e.g. secondary to alcoholism). In adults, skull fractures may remain visible radiologically for years and old fractures mistaken for new injuries.

Direct questioning

Following an acute injury, patients should be asked 'How do you feel now?' Parents of young children should be asked 'How does he seem?' or 'Is she behaving normally?' Symptoms which may occur and which may need to be asked about include: nausea, vomiting, headache, drowsiness, and photophobia. Obviously any injury about the eye should lead to an enquiry about vision and bleeding from the ear to questions about hearing.

Patients often present to A&E departments several weeks after head injury. Symptoms of headache, tiredness, positional vertigo, and difficulties in concentration are very common and may persist for many weeks or months (the post-concussional or post-traumatic syndrome). These should be asked about and their presence or absence noted. This condition must be differentiated from the much rarer chronic subdural haematoma, characterized by a variable level of consciousness. Following a more severe head injury a patient may have behavioural problems and these may need to be asked about from a relative.

Examination

The most important thing to measure in a head-injured patient is their level of consciousness (LOC). This can and should be measured by the Glasgow Coma Score but while this is useful for categorizing patients and monitoring their progress it is not sufficient for the accurate description of a patient's state at a particular point in time. To write:

'*LOC*: GCS = 13'

conveys a certain ammount of information and to write:

'*LOC*: E = 3, M = 6, V = 4, GCS = 13'

conveys a bit more information and also demonstrates that

the doctor knows what he is talking about. Much better, is to describe the patient's state e.g.

'*LOC*:
Appears drowsy,
eyes: open to speech (E = 3)
motor: obeys commands (M = 6)
speech: confused and disorientated (V = 4)
orientation: person √
          place × (no idea where he is)
          time: day   × Tuesday
                 month × December
                 year   × 1976'

or

'Restless and agitated
eyes: open to pain (E = 2)
motor: localizes pain (M = 5) and tries to push away
speech: mumbling, only says "Go away" in answer to any question (V = 3)
GCS = 10'

This gives more information and a clearer picture of the patients state.

The pulse, blood pressure and respiratory rate are the vital signs and must be recorded in any patient with a significant injury. After head injuries these provide the baseline for assessing the changes of raised intracranial pressure.

Wounds, bruises etc. must be noted as described in Chapter 14. Wounds must be inspected. If there is brain coming out of a wound, the patient must have a compound depressed skull fracture with a tear of the dura. Many skull fractures are not visible on radiographs. Therefore, with all wounds that are big enough (even if skull X-rays are being done), the skull should be palpated through the wound and inspected, using a retractor if necessary, to feel or look for evidence of a fracture. This is usually most conveniently done at the time the wound is being sutured and the findings can be recorded in the notes of that procedure but there may be need to do it earlier.

The examination of the head should include a search for

the signs of a basal skull fracture. In particular, the ears should be looked at with an auroscope. There is no need to describe every negative finding, but if a patient has evidence of such an injury, appropriate negative findings should be recorded e.g.

'Bleeding from right ear, EAM full of blood, drum not seen
no bleeding or CSF left ear
Battle's sign negative
no black eyes'

The extent of the neurological examination will obviously depend on the circumstances. A patient who has stood up and hit their head on an open cupboard door, sustaining a laceration but no loss of consciousness and who has had no other symptoms, can almost be regarded as having suffered a scalp laceration rather than a head injury. The following note of the neurological examination would be sufficient:

'Fully conscious, alert and orientated
pupils equal and react to light
walking and using arms normally, CNS grossly intact'

At the other extreme, a patient who has had a severe head injury in a road accident, with much soft tissue damage to the head and face and who is unconscious, obviously has a severe neurological injury. The aim of the neurological examination in these patients is to provide a baseline for the conscious level and limb power, to assess whether the patient has a hemiplegia and to exclude additional neurological injury from spinal trauma. If a patient has no movement of the legs, but moves the arms, they probably have a paraplegia. If they are moving neither arms nor legs to painful stimuli, it is important to test the response to a painful stimulus applied to the head as if this is normal, the patient may have a tetraplegia (see Chapter 20). The initial neurological examination of such a severely head-injured patient should be noted as:

'*LOC*:
comatose, tolerating orophyngeal airway
eyes: closed no reaction to painful stimuli (E = 1)
verbal: none (V = 1)

motor: abnormal flexion left arm and leg, extends right arm and leg to pain (M = 3) GCS = 5
Pupils left normal, reacts normally to light
right dilated sluggish reaction to light
divergent squint'

Examination of the tendon reflexes or the fundi in these patients does not contribute anything to their management at this early stage.

If a patient has such a severe injury that when first seen by the ambulance crew, they had fixed dilated pupils and were not breathing, the question may reasonably be asked whether they are already brain dead and whether resuscitation should be continued. This would be a decision to be made by a senior member of staff but in these cases one may need to look for and record evidence of brainstem function e.g. gag reflex and caloric responses. Dolls eye movements of the eyes should not be tested until cervical spine injury has been excluded!

The full examination of a severely head-injured patient is, of course, more than the examination of the nervous system and head. This and the record keeping for such patients is as described in Chapter 36.

If a patient has symptoms following a head injury, either immediately or if they present after an interval, then a full neurological examination is indicated.

Associated injuries

Patients with a diminished level of consciousness as a result of a head injury will be difficult to assess and in particular it is easy to miss an abdominal injury in a patient who, not only cannot complain of pain, but who may be so deeply unconscious that there is no guarding by the muscles of the abdominal wall. All patients with a significant head injury must be examined fully from head to toe (see Chapter 36). Many will need further investigations to exclude an intra-abdominal injury.

As noted above, an injury in which a moving head strikes a stationary object is likely to cause a neck injury as well as a head injury. All such patients should be assumed to have a neck injury until proved otherwise by normal radiographs and routine physical examination. Patients with a diminished level of consciousness following head injury should also be treated for neck injury. Patients who have been comatose at any time may have aspirated and so the chest must be examined. They may also be unaware of the exact sequence of events leading up to and following the blow to the head and should be examined fully from head to toe. Facial injuries are commonly associated with head injuries.

Other factors to note

Many head injuries occur in patients who have consumed alcohol which may alter behaviour and lower conscious level. This will cause difficulties in assessment. Details of alcohol consumption should be noted and, if possible, a blood or breath alcohol level measured but as noted in Chapter 6 any diminished level of consciousness must be assumed to be due to the head injury and not to the alcohol. A blood alcohol level sufficiently high to cause coma does not exclude an associated severe head injury but, in fact, makes it more likely.

A patient who has suffered an acute head injury should only be discharged to the care of a responsible adult. Their social circumstances should therefore always be enquired about and recorded e.g.

'Will stay at girlfriend's house overnight—discharge—head injury instructions given'

or

'Staying on campsite, no phone, no transport so admit for routine head injury observations'

Notes for patients with head injuries can very usefully be kept on a proforma such as that in Fig. 16.1.

HISTORY

TO BE FILLED IN BY DOCTOR *(If patient unconscious or confused, fill in as much detail as can be obtained)*

SURNAME [ ]   FIRST NAME [ ]   A & E Number [ ]

1		2
History from patient: [ ]	INJURY Date / / hrs	TIME INTERVAL SINCE INJURY:
Other Who?	EXAMINED ON: Date / / hrs	[ ] Days [ ] Hours

Best level of consciousness between injury and arrival in A & E :
Tick one box only

ALERT [ ]

RESPONSE TO VERBAL STIMULI [ ]

RESPONSE TO PAINFUL STIMULI [ ]

UNRESPONSIVE [ ]

See observation chart for Glasgow coma scoring

[3] **DESCRIPTION AND MECHANISM OF INJURIES:** [4]

Hand Dominance
R [ ] L [ ] A [ ] A = Ambidextrous

Occupation (as applicable) [ ]

[5] TICK	[6] SPECIFIC SYMPTOMS: UNCONSCIOUS WHEN SEEN Y [ ]			
		Y=YES	N = NO	U = UNSURE
Driver [ ]				
F/S Passenger [ ]	LOSS OF CONSCIOUSNESS	Y [ ] N [ ] U [ ]		How long?
B/S Passenger [ ]	POST TRAUMATIC AMNESIA	Y [ ] N [ ] U [ ]		How long?
Seatbelt Y [ ] N [ ]	SEIZURE SINCE INJURY	Y [ ] N [ ] U [ ]		Describe:
Motor cyclist [ ]	HEADACHE	Y [ ] N [ ] U [ ]		Describe:
Pillion [ ]	NAUSEA	Y [ ] N [ ] U [ ]		
Pedal cyclist [ ]	VOMITING	Y [ ] N [ ] U [ ]		No of times:
Helmet Y [ ] N [ ]	DROWSY / UNUSUALLY TIRED	Y [ ] N [ ] U [ ]		Comment:
Pedestrian [ ]	VISUAL DISTURBANCE	Y [ ] N [ ] U [ ]		Comment:
Fall [ ]	EVIDENCE OF ALCOHOL	Y [ ] N [ ] U [ ]		Quantity:
Work accident [ ]	CONSUMPTION			Alcohol level: [ ] Time: [ ] hrs
School accident [ ]	EVIDENCE OF DRUG ABUSE	Y [ ] N [ ] U [ ]		Name:
Home accident [ ]	OTHER NEUROLOGICAL			
Assault or NAI [ ]	SYMPTOMS	Y [ ] N [ ] U [ ]		If yes, describe below.
Sport/play [ ]				
Other [ ]				

PRE-EXISTING DISORDERS: *e.g. epilepsy, diabetes, other medical / mental disorder* [7]

NONE [ ]

UNKNOWN [ ]

TETANUS STATE: COVERED [ ]   NEEDS BOOSTER [ ]   NEEDS COURSE [ ]   NOT KNOWN [ ] [8]

DRUG THERAPY: [9]	**DRUG ALLERGIES:** [10]
NONE [ ]	NONE [ ]
UNKNOWN [ ]	UNKNOWN [ ]

Staff are advised to consult the A&E Head Injury Proforma Guide (HIPG/1993)

Fig. 16.1 • Proforma for recording information on head-injured patients. (© Quest, A&E Proforma Group, and reproduced by permission.)

EXAMINATION

Illustrate injuries with appropriate measurements of lacerations and bruises in cms: **NO LACERATIONS:** ☐ **NO BRUISES:** ☐ [1]

				[2] Comments:	[4]
SUSPICION OF COMPOUND SKULL FRACTURE OR PENETRATING INJURY	Y ☐	N ☐			
EVIDENCE OF BASAL SKULL FRACTURE	Y ☐	N ☐			
CSF LEAK FROM NOSE / EAR	Y ☐	N ☐			

EVIDENCE OF INJURY TO NECK   Y ☐   N ☐ [3]

NEUROLOGICAL EXAMINATION

Doctor MUST document responsiveness, pupil and limb movement responses in boxes 1, 2 & 3 on observation chart opposite.

ORIENTATED IN: TIME Y ☐   N ☐   PLACE Y ☐   N ☐   PERSON Y ☐   N ☐ [5]

				[6]
EVIDENCE OF DYSPHASIA	Y ☐ N ☐	HEARING LOSS / FACIAL WEAKNESS	Y ☐ N ☐	
INAPPROPRIATE / ABNORMAL BEHAVIOUR	Y ☐ N ☐	EVIDENCE OF ABNORMAL GAIT	Y ☐ N ☐	
LOSS OF VISION / ABNORMAL EYE MOVEMENT	Y ☐ N ☐	EVIDENCE OF ABNORMAL FINE LIMB MOVEMENT	Y ☐ N ☐	

TREATMENT

INVESTIGATIONS AND RESULTS: [7]

X-RAY: SKULL Y ☐ N ☐   NECK   Y ☐ N ☐

REASON FOR SKULL X-RAY ☐

Findings:

Other investigations:

DIAGNOSIS: *tick as appropriate*

☐ Minor HI, fully orientated, no evidence of skull fracture (on clinical or radiological grounds)

☐ Minor HI, fully orientated, with skull fracture

☐ Disorientated / drowsy

☐ Difficult to assess

☐ Moderate / severe head injury

☐ Other diagnosis / injury

MANAGEMENT: *Tick as appropriate:* [9]

Home with head injury instructions ☐

Name of responsible person at home ☐

Request opinion of ☐

Admit to short stay ward ☐

Admit to other ward ☐

Reason for admission ☐

Other treatment, eg sutures, tetanus and antibiotics:

Head injury instructions explained and given   Y ☐   N ☐

Doctors signature:

HI/03   © GULLAN & WALLACE 1992   HIPAN/93

Examples of notes on head injury

History (from patient, father, and ambulance crew):
Cycling down hill, lost control, wheel hit kerb, flew over handlebars head and right shoulder hit the pavement. (Not wearing helmet.) Was unconscious for about 2 mins.
When ambulance arrived was sitting up, talking but confused, walked into ambulance. Vomited × 1 in ambulance.
Patients next memory is of being in the ambulance (i.e. PTA approx 10–15 mins.)
Now has headache all over. No nausea. No pain anywhere else. No neck pain.

PMH:
Nil, drugs nil, allergies nil, tetanus status — preschool booster 4 years ago.

O/E:
Fit child, fully alert and orientated
P 96 BP 105/65 RR 22
5 cm ragged laceration transverse, Right frontal region, just above the hairline.
PERL, fundi not examined, full eye movements, no diplopia
Power L = R = strong
Reflexes L = R = brisk
Plantars ↓ ↓
Neck no tenderness, full ROM (painless)
No sign trauma to right shoulder, full painless ROM
No evidence of other injury
Spine Chest — clear, no pain on springing ribs, Abdo soft, Pelvis √ Legs √ √ normal gait.

Skull: XR — NBI.

Diagnosis: Minor head injury (PTA poss 15 mins) with laceration.

Plan:
Suture
Head injury instruction sheet
Advised paracetamol
To see GP for sutures out 7/7
Advised to wear cycle helmet.

Theatre:
1% lignocaine
Wound cleaned, edges trimmed, skull seen and palpated, no obvious fracture
6 × 3/0 ethilon sutures no tension.

or

History:
5/7 ago locked out of house, stood on dustbin to try to get in window. Fell off, hit head on gravel path (left parietal region). Full memory of all events. Didn't seek medical help.
Since then continuous headaches, all over, worst at site of injury, worse as day goes on, not improving but not getting worse.
Not helped by paracetamol

DQ:
No nausea or vomiting but generally tired.
Can't concentrate for more than ½ hour.
2 episodes of vertigo getting in and out of bed, lasted a few seconds.

PMH:
Mild asthma: salbutamol inhaler prn—usually about once a fortnight. Never needed admission or steroids.
Nil else

O/E:
P 78 SR, BP 130/80.
Fully alert and orientated.
Pupils equal and react to light.
Fundi normal.
Full eye movements, no diplopia, 2 or 3 beats of nystagmus to both left and right.
V motor and sensory normal.
VII no facial weakness.
VII grossly normal, EAMs normal.
Cranials IX—XII normal.

Limbs:
Power left = right = strong in all groups.
Sensation grossly intact in all 4 limbs.

Reflexes:

	Right	Left
BJ	++	++
TJ	++	++
SJ	++	++
KJ	++	++
AJ	+	+
Pl	↓	↓

Normal gait
Normal co-ordination
Diagnosis: Post-traumatic syndrome.

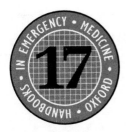

CHAPTER 17

Face injury

Black eye

A black eye is usually the result of a direct injury to the eye, often a punch. It is important to differentiate between an uncomplicated periorbital haematoma and an underlying fracture of the zygoma or orbital floor. One should also exclude an injury to the eye itself. Features of a fractured zygoma which must be looked for are:

- A palpable step in the orbital rim.
- Displacement of the zygoma (often difficult to detect initially because of soft tissue swelling).
- A lateral subconjunctival haemorrhage without a posterior limit.
- Tenderness over the zygomatico-frontal suture.
- Surgical emphysema of the orbit.
- If the zygomatic arch is fractured, it will be tender and there may be interference with jaw opening (which may be confused with a mandibular condyle injury).

Signs of an orbital floor (blow-out) fracture include:

- Diminished and possibly painful eye movement and diplopia (especially on upward gaze).
- Anaesthesia in the area supplied by the infraorbital and superior dental nerves.

Bilateral black eyes in the absence of a local injury may signify a basal skull fracture (see head injuries, Chapter 16).

Examples of notes on a black eye

O/E:
Right black eye
vision 6/6 6/6
full ROM eyes, no diplopia
no steps, tenderness, numbness of cheek
clinically NBI.

or

O/E:
Right black eye
lateral subconjunctival haemorrhage
vision 6/6 6/6
tender step infraorbital rim
tender Z–F suture
diplopia on upward gaze
numbness cheek.
clinically # zygoma/blow-out
X-ray:

Nose injuries

History

Those who most often break their nose (e.g. fighters and rugby players) may well have broken their nose before. Enquire about this and, if they have broken it before and the nose appears bent, ask them if it is any more bent now than it was before this most recent injury (a recent photograph may help). Previous nasal surgery or other problems (e.g. septal deviation) is obviously of relevance. Ask also if the nose bled when they injured it as the nose which did not bleed is almost certainly not broken. Ask whether they can breathe normally through the nose. If the nose is deviated but there is no airway problem then the only indication for treatment is to improve the appearance. Ask the patient (and, on occasion the patient's partner) if they want the nose to be straightened and also ask about past medical problems.

There is no point asking the patient to return for treatment if they are happy with the shape of the nose or if general anaesthesia for a cosmetic operation would be contra-indicated because of other medical problems.

Examination

It is important to establish:

1. Is the nose straight? This may be difficult to judge initially because of soft tissue swelling. If in doubt, the patient should be reviewed when the swelling is less in, say, five days.
2. Is the nasal septum midline and is there a septal haematoma?
3. Is the airway patent through each nostril?

Associated injuries

Nasal injuries may be associated with other facial injuries, especially zygomatic fractures (see above). These should be looked for.

Examples of notes on nose injuries

History:
Rugby injury, ran into post and injured nose. No other injury.
PMH: No previous nose injuries/problems.
O/E:
Nose bruised, minimally deviated towards right, small abrasion bridge of nose
no septal haematoma
septum midline
airway patent through each nostril
no evidence # zygoma.
Diagnosis: # nose, slight displacement only.
Plan:
Happy with shape
no treatment required
return within 5 days if changes mind and wants treatment.

or

O/E:
Nose bent towards left
septum deviated to right with decreased airway right nostril
no septal haematoma
Diagnosis: # nose.
Plan: Refer next ENT clinic.

Dental injuries

Terminology

Doctors usually have very little training in, and see very few dental problems. An exception is dental injuries. Patients frequently attend an A&E department rather than a dentist because these are acute problems, often occurring out of hours and are frequently associated with other injuries. In view of their poor education on dental matters, doctors often lack the terminology to describe dental problems. It is not necessary to know all the terms used by dentists but it is essential to know enough to accurately describe the injuries and other problems which they encounter, accurately both in the notes and to any faciomaxillary surgeon or dentist to whom they refer the patient.

A full set of permanent teeth is shown diagramatically as:

8	7	6	5	4	3	2	1	1	2	3	4	5	6	7	8
8	7	6	5	4	3	2	1	1	2	3	4	5	6	7	8

and individual teeth are represented and described as e.g.

 2 |—upper right 2

⌈ 67—lower left 6 and 7

Teeth can also be described as e.g.

upper left central incisor
lower right first premolar

A full set of deciduous teeth is shown diagramatically as:

e	d	c	b	a	a	b	c	d	e
e	d	c	b	a	a	b	c	d	e

and individual teeth are described in a similar way to adult teeth.

A premolar or molar tooth has five exposed surfaces:

Proximal: nearest to the TM joint
Distal: furthest from the TM joint
Buccal: the side nearest the cheek
Lingual: the side nearest the tongue
Occlusal: the part against which one chews

History

When patients arrive in A&E the name and address of their general medical practitioner will be noted routinely by the reception staff. If a patient has dental problems it may be necessary to note the name of the patient's general dental practitioner, especially if the patient is going to be referred to them for follow-up or definitive treatment.

In children with dental injuries one needs to establish whether the injuries are to deciduous or permanent teeth.

In anyone who has lost teeth or who has bits of denture missing, it is important to ascertain that none was inhaled.

When enquiring about past history there is no need to go into great detail about previous dental problems (which one may not even understand!) but it is important to know whether the patient has any (expensive) bridges or crowns among the injured teeth.

Example of notes on dental injuries

History:
In cricket nets this p.m. Hit in mouth by cricket ball and injured teeth. No crowns/bridges.
O/E:

1 ⌐ 1 knocked out

alveolar fracture with loosening of 2 ⌐ 3
 1 ⌐ chipped
 3 ⌐ missing (long-standing).

Mandibular injuries

History

Apart from the standard questions concerning mechanism of injury etc., one important question to ask the patient is whether their dental occlusion feels right (ask 'When you bite, do your teeth seem to be in the right place?'). If the occlusion is wrong there is almost certainly an injury to either the upper or lower jaw.

Examination

Severe mandibular fractures may cause airway problems. This is discussed in Chapter 36. The signs of a mandibular fracture are:

Look:
(at the face and inside the mouth)
malocclusion
bruising under the tongue
laceration of the mucosa
loose teeth
possible visible step in the jaw.

Feel:
Tenderness (NB palpate the whole mandible as it is very common to have more than one fracture in the mandible e.g. one angle and the condyle on the opposite side or both condyles).

Move:
Jaw movements (both opening and movement from side to side) will be painful and possibly limited. Jaw opening is probably best measured by the separation of the teeth at full opening. Crepitus may be noted.

Special tests:
Anaesthesia in the region supplied by the mental nerve should be looked for and noted if present.
Stressing the mandible. Squeezing the two angles of the mandible will cause pain at a fracture site and if the patient has his mouth open, pressure on the chin will cause pain in the condlylar region if the patient has a fracture there.

Examples of notes on jaw injuries

History:
Injured jaw in rugby scrum yesterday. Exact mechanism uncertain, able to finish game. Can eat normally. Teeth feel they are in the right position.
Examination:
Some bruising and slight tenderness left temporomandibular joint.
Occlusion normal. No bruising etc. inside mouth.
Full painless ROM TM joints. No pain on biting or springing of mandible.
Diagnosis: Bruising over left TM joint.

or

History:
Assaulted by husband who punched her once on left side of jaw. Fell backwards landing on a chair. No loss of consciousness. No other injury. Husband never assaulted her before. Has drunk about 1½ pints lager and one gin.
Occlusion wrong.
O/E:
Fully conscious and alert but obviously in pain.
Drooling blood stained saliva from mouth. Difficulty in speaking.
Bruising right side of chin.
Mucosal tear and ? step between 23‾
Tender ++ over anterior right mandible. also slightly tender left condyle.
Jaw movements reduced — can only open mouth about 2 cm.
Sensation normal
Diagnosis:
Clinically # body mandible on right, ? left condyle.
X-ray:

Middle third facial fractures

Fractures of the middle third of the face are caused by major forces and the patient may have other injuries. These fractures can cause severe airway problems, especially if the patient has a diminished level of consciousness as a result of an associated head injury. These patients must be managed as patients with major injuries as described in Chapter 36. The main sign is mobility of the facial skeleton which can be elicited by pushing on the hard palette. If there is movement the patient has a middle third fracture. Various tests have been described to differentiate between the three main types of fracture (Le Fort I, II, and III). These determine whether it is just the hard palette which moves (Le Fort I), whether the central part of the facial skeleton moves (Le Fort II) or whether the whole facial skeleton moves in relation to the skull (Le Fort III). Variations do occur (e.g. a Le Fort II on the left and both a Le Fort II and III on the right) and these tests are not always conclusive. The A&E doctor's responsibility is to determine that a fracture exists and the facio-maxillary surgeon can determine its type.

Le Fort II and III fractures may involve the cribriform plate and so may be associated with cerebrospinal fluid rhinorrhoea. This should be noted if it is seen but in the first few hours after injury it is mixed with blood and is usually impossible to differentiate from a pure epistaxis.

Patients with evidence of severe injury to the face should have notes which include such lines as:

'Bilateral black eyes and severe soft tissue swelling of face — palette mobile
Diagnosis: fracture middle third'.

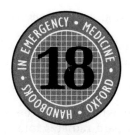

CHAPTER 18

Cervical spine injury

History

As with all injuries it is important to try to understand the forces involved in a neck injury. Many such injuries occur in road accidents and details of how to assess these can be found in Chapter 37. Clearly a patient who turned quickly and developed severe neck pain is unlikely to have a significant bony injury whereas the patient involved in a high velocity injury or who falls down stairs is greatly at risk of a fracture. It is important to try to differentiate between hyperflexion and hyperextension injuries, with or without rotation, as each may produce a specific pattern of damage. Vertical loading of the spine may cause burst fractures and the patient with a sudden onset of pain while doing doing heavy work may have an avulsion fracture of a spinous process (clay shovellers' fracture).

Past medical history

The past medical history may occasionally be of vital importance in the assessment of a cervical spine injury. The spine with metastatic bony deposits may fracture with minimal trauma, which would not be expected to injure a normal spine, as may the rigid spine of ankylosing spondylitis. This latter fracture will behave like a long bone fracture and will almost always be unstable. Many patients have pre-existing neck pain or stiffness due to degenerative or intervertebral disc disease in their neck. This will be exacerbated by an injury and uncommonly pre-existing neurological problems (e.g. multiple sclerosis) may cause confusion in the assessment of these injuries.

Symptoms

Most patients with neck injuries present with pain in the neck. It is important to ask whether this pain radiates into the shoulders and arms or into the head. If pain radiates into the arms it is important to know exactly how far down the arm and into which fingers it goes. One should also ask about neurological symptoms such as weakness, numbness, and paraesthesiae; and the precise location of any parasthesiae should be noted and related to the dermatomes of the upper limb (see Fig. 18.1). If a patient has any symptoms in the legs one should ask about bladder function.

Examination

The examination of the neck can be summarized as

- Look
- Feel
- Move
- Neurological examination

If a patient has been involved in a high velocity accident, the ambulance personnel will often place the patient in a firm collar as a routine. On arrival in A&E the patient should be asked if they have any neck pain. If they are fully conscious and say they have no pain the collar can be removed and the examination can continue as normal. If, however, they complain of pain or are difficult to assess because of other injuries or intoxication, a full examination should wait until the patient has been X-rayed. When a patient returns from the X-ray department with normal films it is easy to forget the physical examination. It is important that this does not happen.

Fig. 18.1 • The dermatomes of the body.

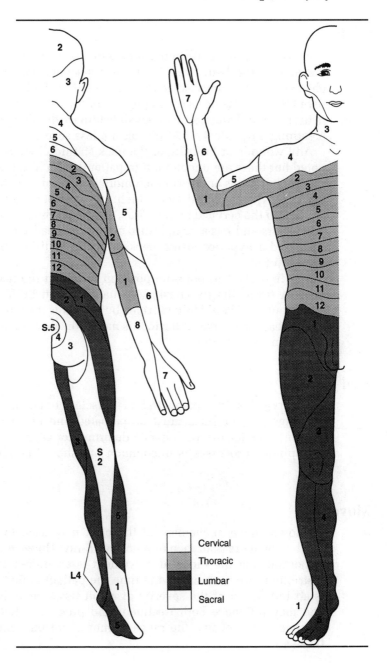

Look

A complete spinal cord injury may often be diagnosed from the end of the bed, even in the unconscious patient, by observing such things as lack of movement in the legs compared to the arms or face; the posture of the arms; priapism in the male; and intercostal paralysis leading to diaphragmatic breathing only. Most neck injuries are less severe.

Any wounds or bruising of the neck should obviously be noted but these are uncommon in patients with blunt cervical spine injuries and it is much more important to note the marks on the head and face which will indicate the forces applied to the cervical spine. Thus, a patient who has fallen downstairs and has a large bruise on the forehead will have sustained a hyperextension neck injury in addition to any head injury.

It is important to note the position in which the neck is held. A torticollis (wryneck) is usually caused by muscle spasm but this should be confirmed by palpating the muscles. In the absence of spasm, torticollis may indicate a unilateral facet joint dislocation.

Feel

The cervical spine, paravertebral muscles, trapezius, and sternomastoid muscles must be palpated and any tenderness must be localized. Palpable deformity or gaps between the spinous processes is uncommon but should be looked for.

Move

As noted above, movement of the neck may need to wait until after the reassurance of a normal X-ray. However, it is important that the range of movement is examined as the restriction of movement at the time the patient is first seen is an indication of the severity of a soft tissue neck injury and may influence both treatment and prognosis. Records must include not just the range of movement but whether these are painful.

The movements of the cervical spine are:

- Flexion and extension.
- Lateral flexion to left and right.
- Rotation to left and right.

Movements can be measured in degrees but this can be difficult to estimate. For practical purposes, immediately after an injury, it is sufficient to estimate the range of movement as a percentage of the normal range which you would expect in a patient of similar age and build.

For a more accurate description of the range of neck flexion (e.g. for follow-up or for medicolegal purposes) one can measure the distance between the chin and the chest wall on full neck flexion and lateral flexion can be measured as the distance between the ear and the shoulder (ensure that the patient does not elevate the shoulder). A normal range of movement can be illustrated diagramatically as:

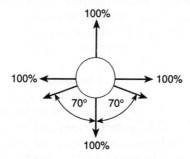

Neurological examination

An injury of the cervical spine may injure the spinal cord, nerve roots, or both. In addition, the multiply-injured patient may have other neurological injuries, especially of the brachial plexus. On occasion patients may have a pre-existing neurological problem to confuse the picture. It is important that every doctor developes an examination technique to identify nerve root and cord injuries.

In the patient with a neck injury who walks into the A&E department and has no complaints of leg problems, the neurological examination can be confined to the arms. One needs to test muscle power and sensation related to each nerve root from C5 to T1.

A basic initial examination can consist of examining power in:

Shoulder abduction	to test C5
Elbow flexion	to test C6
Elbow extension	to test C7
Finger flexion	to test C8
Intrinsic muscles of hand	to test T1

but if weakness is discovered in any muscle, other muscles supplied by the same nerve root should be tested. Thus, if the power in biceps (C5,6), used as a screening test to exclude a C6 root injury is reduced then wrist extension (C6,7) should be tested too.

Muscle power should be expressed according to the Medical Research Council grading (Table 18.1). It is important to differentiate between true weakness due to nerve injury and lack of strength because contraction of the muscle causes pain in the neck. Muscles should be palpated while testing power to feel the contraction.

Sensation should be tested in both arms and any loss of or alteration in sensation related to dermatomes (Fig. 18.1). Sensory loss in one dermatome (especially if associated with weakness of the muscles supplied by the same nerve root) is likely to indicate a root injury whereas numbness in a glove distribution is unlikely to be significant.

The tendon reflexes in the arms should be elicited; the root distribution of these is shown in Table 18.2.

Table 18.1 • Medical Research Council grading of muscle power

0	No contraction
1	Flicker or trace of contraction
2	Active movement with gravity eliminated
3	Active movement against gravity
4	Active movement against gravity and resistance
5	Normal power

Table 18.2 • Nerve supply of tendon reflexes

Biceps jerk	(BJ)	C5,6
Triceps jerk	(TJ)	C7
Supinator jerk	(SJ)	C6
Knee jerk	(KJ)	L3,4
Ankle jerk	(AJ)	S1,2

Associated injuries

The common association of head injuries and neck injuries has been discussed. It is usually the neck injury which is overlooked and it is unlikely that a patient who presents with a neck injury will have an occult head injury. There is also an association between neck and shoulder injuries and it is frequently assumed that shoulder pain following a neck injury is referred from the neck. This may be so but the patient with shoulder pain following an accident needs an examination of the shoulder (see Chapter 23).

Examples of notes on neck injuries

History:
Car driver. Wearing seatbelt. No head restraints.
stationary at roundabout when hit from behind by another car. Possibly 20 mph impact.
Not KO'd, Remembers whole incident. Head did not hit windscreen. Got out of car unaided but immediately felt pain in neck and sat down. No other injury.
Now has pain in neck, radiates into left shoulder. No weakness, numbness or paraesthesiae arms or legs.
PMH: Nil significant.
O/E:
In firm collar (put on by ambulance personnel)—not removed, points to left side of neck as site of pain.
Power in arms: left = right = strong in all groups except shoulder abduction on left weak ($^4/_5$) because of pain in neck. Resisted elbow flexion also causes pain.

Sensation: normal in both upper limbs.
Reflexes: left = right = brisk.
Shoulders: no tenderness, full painless ROM.
Provisional diagnosis: probable neck sprain but exclude a fracture.
X-ray: NBI.
Collar removed, no vertebral tenderness, tender left trapezius. Full ROM but pain on rotation to right.
Diagnosis: minor neck sprain.

or

Tripped on loose carpet and fell down 8 stairs 3/7 ago. Hit back of head but not KO'd. Did not seek medical help. Since then pain in neck radiating to finger tips right hand—all the fingers (not thumb). Also paraesthesiae lower arm and weakness right hand.
PMH:
Mild hypertension 4 years on bendrofluazide 5 mg od 'whiplash' injury 2 years ago XR—NBI, off work 2/52 fully better in 3/12. No other neck problems.
O/E:
Healing abrasion occiput, no swelling.
Tender C5—T2.
ROM: Lateral flexion and rotation to left exacerbate paraesthesiae.
Power:

	Right	Left
shoulder abduction	4/5 (painful)	5/5
elbow flexion	5/5	5/5
elbow extension	5/5	5/5
grip	4/5	5/5
abd. dig. min.	3/5	5/5
interossei	3/5	5/5
opponens	3/5	5/5

Reflexes:

	Right	Left
BJ	++	++
TJ	++	++
SJ	++	++

Sensation: Normal on left, alteration of sensation medial side arm and forearm.

Diagnosis: Neck injury with T1 root lesion.

X-ray:

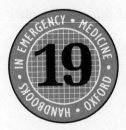

CHAPTER 19

Thoracic and lumbar injuries

When talking to someone who presents with a back injury or back pain it is wise at an early stage in taking the history to ask them to point to the site of the pain. It is very common for patients who say they have injured their back to have an injury of the posterior chest wall or loin rather than the spine. This will affect the way you approach the history and examination and early identification of the injured area will speed the consultation.

History

As with all other areas of the body, an accurate history will give valuable pointers to the type and severity of the injury. A hyperflexion injury will cause one or more wedge fractures whereas a blow to the back commonly causes a fracture of a transverse process. A patient who bends down and gets severe back pain will not have a bony injury (unless he or she is at risk of a pathological fracture) but will have a soft tissue problem (commonly a prolapsed intervertebral disc).

The symptom of pain should be explored further. Pain made worse by coughing or sneezing indicates dural irritation, commonly due to a prolapsed intervertebral disc. If there is referred pain into the legs, this will usually be volunteered by the patient but one should enquire how far down and into which part of the leg it goes. Weakness, paraesthesiae and numbness should be asked about and related to dermatomes. Bladder symptoms should be enquired about in the patient who presents after an interval (there is no point asking about difficulty in micturition in a patient who only injured himself half an hour earlier).

A patient with a back injury or back pain is likely to have been told to undress and lie on a trolley so they can be properly examined. It is easy for a doctor seeing such a patient to assume they have been brought in supine by the ambulance service. It is useful to ask whether they have walked since the accident. If they have walked, the injury is unlikely to be very severe and the patient can be stood or sat up to have their back fully examined. The patient who has suffered significant forces and has not walked since the accident will need to be 'log-rolled' for their back to be examined until radiographs demonstrate the absence of a serious fracture.

As with cervical spine injuries, the patient with a history of malignancy may suffer a pathological fracture with minimal trauma. The most common cause of pathological fracture in the lumbar spine is osteoporosis, either post-menopausal or caused by steroid therapy. This should be noted and communicated to the general practitioner as the patient may need investigation and possibly treatment for osteoporosis. Previous back injuries, pain, and other problems must of course be noted.

Examination
Look

If the patient walks into the A&E department they can be examined standing up and the normal curves of the spine should be noted. Kyphosis, scoliosis, or an increase in the normal lumbar lordosis should be noted. The shape of any scoliolis can be described as e.g. 'convex/concave to left/right'. These curves are more difficult to see in the patient who is lying down and who has been 'log rolled' on to their side but any sharp angulation suggestive of a fracture should be noted.

Feel

The whole spine needs to be palpated and the spinal level of maximum tenderness noted, and whether the tenderness is midline as one would expect with a fracture of the spine or to one side, which may be more suggestive of a fracture of the transverse process. While palpating each spinous process the gaps between them should be palpated, a large gap, indicating a tear in the interspinous ligament, is indicative of an unstable injury.

Move

Whether one can test back movements will depend on the severity of the injury. The back has the same six movements as the neck but measuring them accurately is not easy.

An appropriate way of estimating forward flexion of the spine is to ask the patient to touch their toes and then to measure the distance of the finger tips from the floor. Most patients have an idea how far they can normally bend forward and this can be stated for comparison e.g. '*flexion*: fingers to 8 cm from floor, normally can touch toes'. This is sufficient for the assessment and follow-up of flexion in the acutely injured back but as an absolute measure flexion it is very inaccurate, as the ability to touch ones toes is a composite movement of hips and back. It is possible for a patient with an ankylosed spine to touch their toes if they have sufficient flexibility of the hips. This can be partially assessed by watching the patient as they bend forward and ensuring that the normal lordosis is reversed. For example one can note:

'*flexion*: fingers to lower pole patella, lordosis not abolished'

This method is probably sufficient for the acutely injured patient but for an accurate measurement of back flexion one should measure the increased in length of the spine which occurs in flexion.

Lateral flexion can be measured by measuring the position of the finger tips related to the patella e.g.

'*lateral flexion*:
to right fingers 10 cm below lower pole patella
to left 2 cm above upper pole patella.

When measuring rotation, the pelvis should be held still and the patient asked to rotate to left and right. It is measured by the angle between the shoulders and the pelvis.

Extension is the most difficult movement to measure accurately. It should be measured in degrees but in practice it is best measured as a percentage of what one would expect to find in a patient of similar age and build.

Neurological examination

In the patient with a lower back injury or with acute back pain who walks into the A&E department one is primarily interested in examining the patient to exclude injuries to nerve roots. The initial examination should consist of examining:

Hip flexion	to test L2,3
Knee extension	to test L3,4
Ankle dorsiflexion	to test L4,5
Big toe dorsiflexion	to test L5
Ankle plantar flexion	to test S1,2

Additional movements can be tested if any of these are weak or difficult to test because of pain. The dermatomes are shown in Fig. 18.1 and sensation must be tested within each dermatome.

The root origin of the tendon reflexes is shown in Table 18.2. It is not normally necessary to test sacral sensation and anal tone in every patient with a back injury or back pain but it should be part of the examination in anybody with any possibility of injury to sacral cord or roots e.g. patients with severe pain, patients with sacral fractures, and patients with urinary symptoms.

Other tests

Straight leg-raising should be measured in all patients with acute back pain and if relevant the sciatic stretch test can be performed. In patients with suspected injuries to the upper nerve roots, the femoral stretch test should be done.

If the patient is mobile, the gait should be noted (see Chapter 27). If the patient is immobile because of pain, some comment can be made in the notes about their mobility in bed e.g. can they sit up, roll over unaided.

Because of the association betwen injuries to the transverse processes and the kidney, any patient with a fracture of the transverse process should have the urine examined to exclude haematuria and the result noted.

Examples of notes on thoracic or lumbar injuries

History:

1 hr ago.

Tripped on loose carpet and fell down 3 steps, landing on lower back. No other injuries.

Walked a few steps into ambulance and then into A&E.

Now severe pain back (points to lumbar spine and left loin).

No radiation of pain.

PMH: Nil significant. No medication.

O/E:

In pain but able to move about the bed.

No deformity.

Some bruising and a red mark over L 1–3 and left paravertebral muscles.

Tender whole of lumbar spine but maximally tender to the over bruised area.

Power left = right = strong in all groups.

sensation intact both sides L 1–S 1

Reflexes:

	Right	Left
KJ	++	++
AJ	++	++
Pl	↓	↓

Movements not examined because of pain.

Assessment: ? fracture transverse process on left.

X-ray lumbar spine: confirms # left TP L1 and ? L2.

Urine clear (passed urine normally).

Admit for analgesia/mobilization.

or

History:

This p.m. at work went to pick up object from floor and back 'went' sudden pain lower back radiating into left foot as far as ankle. Pain worse if coughs.

Managed to straighten up and walk to first aid room. First aider
brought him here in works' van.
No weakness or paraesthesiae.
PMH:
tibia and fibula (M/C crash) 5 years ago. Nil else. No back problems.
Allergic to aspirin (face swells).
O/E:
Stands with increased lordosis.
Tender L5.
All back movements greatly reduced by pain (on flexion finger tips to knees only).
Power:

	Right	Left
Hip flexion		
extension		
Knee flexion	Right = left = strong	
extension		
Ankle dorsiflexion		
plantarflexion	5/5	4/5
Toe flexion	5/5	3/5

Sensation:	normal	decreased lateral border and little toe

Reflexes: KJ	++	++
AJ	+	−
Pl	↓	↓

SLR:	50°	30°

Gait: Walks very slowly with back held very stiffly. Difficulty getting off bed unaided.
Diagnosis: Prolapsed intervertebral disc at S1.

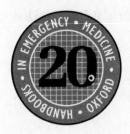

CHAPTER 20

Spinal cord injury

If a patient has a spinal cord injury whether from trauma or, less commonly in an A&E setting, from a non-traumatic cause, such as an acute cord compression or a vascular problem, it is important to document the level and to determine whether the injury is complete or incomplete. By convention, the level of a cord injury is the level of the last intact segment. Thus, a patient with who can flex his or her elbows actively but who cannot extend them has a C6 spinal cord injury whereas the patient who can abduct the shoulders but who has no elbow movement has a C5 injury. Any patient in whom cord problems are suspected must have a full neurological examination including examination of the anal tone and sacral sensation. If this is intact, the spinal cord lesion is not complete. If a patient does have a partial spinal cord lesion, they must have a very detailed examination including all sensory modalities to define the injury. These partial cord syndromes are rare in A&E practice but a central cord syndrome with dissociated sensory loss may occur in neck injury without bony injury and the Brown-Séquard syndrome may occur following a stab wound to the cord.

The patient with a spinal cord injury may be hypotensive because of the injury to the sympathetic nerves, and patients with high cord injuries causing intercostal muscle paralysis are at risk of respiratory failure especially if there is an associated chest injury. The pulse, blood pressure, and respiratory rate should be measured routinely and an assessment made of respiratory function.

Associated injuries

A cervical cord injury occurring in a rugby scrum is unlikely to be associated with any other significant injury but the same injury caused by a road accident may be one of a series of injuries. Unfortunately, these may be difficult to diagnose if the patient is tetraplegic and has no sensation below the level of the neck injury. Therefore, a very careful head to toe examination must always be done and documented (see Chapter 36) and the examination of the abdomen augmented by other procedures (computerized tonography, ultrasound, or peritoneal lavage) to exclude an occult abdominal injury.

Treatment

Patients with cervical spine injuries are greatly at risk of any neurological lesion being worsened by movement. Patients with spinal cord injuries are prone to many complications (e.g. pressure sores and urinary tract infections), which may, on occasion, start in A&E. Patient care must be scrupulous and this made obvious in the notes.

Example of notes on spinal cord injury

History:
Rugby prop forward. Set scrum collapsed. Acute pain in neck. Unable to move. Not KO'd.
Ambulance found unable to move legs. Applied a firm collar and brought him here.
Now pain in neck, says he can't feel his feet.
Past history: nil, Drugs: nil, Allergies: nil.
O/E:
P 105, BP 100/65, RR 25, GCS 15.
Fully alert and orientated, anxious. Not pale or sweaty. Priapism.
In firm collar, sandbags/tape added. Cervical spine not examined.
Airway: clear.

Breathing:
no movement of intercostals, diaphragmatic breathing only.
Trachea central, chest clear. O_2 given by mask.
Circulation: P & BP as above, normal capillary return IVI
inserted.
Arms held flexed, can't extend elbows.
Power:

shoulder abduction	5/5	5/5
elbow flexion	5/5	5/5
extension	0	0
wrist extension	4/5	4/5
flexion	0	0
finger flexion	0	0
extension	0	0
intrinsics	0	0

No power in legs
Sensation: present over shoulder and down lateral side of
both arms to thumbs (C5/6).
No sensation rest of hand, medial side of arm, chest, abdomen
or legs.
Reflexes:

	Right	Left
BJ	++	++
TJ	−	−
SJ	+	+
KJ	−	−
AJ	−	−
Pl	−	−
Abdo	−	−

Head to toe examination: . . .
Log-rolled:
No marks, bruising,
spine normal, no steps etc.
No sensation on back
No sacral sensation, PR: no anal tone, rectum empty, prostate
normal.
Gravel cleared from under him, laid on a fleece
Diagnosis: Cervical cord injury C6, no evidence other injury.
X-ray: Cervical spine.
Chest.

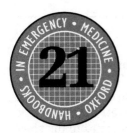

CHAPTER 21

Chest injury

History

It is important to differentiate between: (1) low velocity injury which is likely to cause an injury to the chest wall only; (2) a more severe crushing injury which may cause asphyxia in addition to the chest injury; and (3) the high velocity injury which may damage mediastinal structures and cause significant pulmonary contusion. With a low velocity injury the exact mechanism will differentiate between the injury which is unlikely to have caused more than a single rib fracture (which may not even require an X-ray) and the rather greater force which may have caused multiple rib fractures.

Patients will usually be in pain, especially on inspiration and the decision to admit the patient depends largely on the severity of pain rather than on whether one or more rib fractures are visible on an X-ray. The pain severity should therefore be assessed. Patients also need to be asked about shortness of breath and haemoptysis. If the injury is already some days old, a complicating chest infection may need to be excluded by asking about cough and sputum production. Patients with chest injuries should also always be asked about their past medical history and smoking habits. In a patient with severe chronic obstructive airways disease or other problems, a single rib fracture may prove fatal and such a patient will need admission to hospital whereas a fitter patient may not even seek medical help.

Examination

In a patient who has minor marks on the chest wall but in whom a significant chest wall injury is not suspected, 'springing' the chest wall from side to side and front to back, if painless, will exclude a serious chest wall injury.

Blunt chest trauma will usually cause injuries to the chest wall and the underlying pleural cavities and lungs. Significant cardiac injury is rare although the possibility in a high velocity injury must always be considered as it must in a penetrating injury anywhere near the mediastinum. The heart and cardiovascular system should be examined as well as the respiratory system in all cases of chest trauma. A cardiac murmur in a previously fit young patient following a chest injury may be caused by a traumatic valvular lesion.

The examination of the chest can be summarized as:

Evidence of injury
Bruising, wounds
Tenderness
Surgical emphysema
Paradoxical respiration (flail segment)
Palpable crepitus
Work of breathing
Respiratory rate
Use of accessory muscles
Mechanics of breathing
Chest movement
Air entry
Breath sounds
Tracheal position
Percussion
Effects of breathing
Cyanosis
Level of consciousness (it must not be forgotten that a lowered level of consciousness may be caused by hypoxia or blood loss as well as by a head injury)
Oxygen saturation (measured by pulse oximeter)
Evidence of blood loss
Pulse

Blood pressure
Capillary return
Colour
Peripheral skin temperature
Examination of the heart
Heart sounds
Jugular venous pressure (especially for cardiac tamponade)
Femoral pulse (if absent, consider ruptured aorta)

Associated injuries

The chest is commonly injured in road traffic accidents
when it can frequently occur with abdominal, thoracic spine,
and other injuries. In particular, fractures are associated with
liver, spleen, or (less commonly) renal injuries. Fractures of
the first rib are uncommon but are usually caused by major
forces which may also cause axillary artery and brachial
plexus injuries. The arterial and nerve supplies to the arm
should be examined in any patient with this injury (see
Chapter 25). In expiration, the diaphragm may come as high
as the 4th intercostal space and any penetrating wound below this level may have entered the abdominal cavity. Examination of the abdomen must be performed in patients
with penetrating chest trauma.

Note keeping

In all patients who have sustained significant trauma it is
important to note the pulse, blood pressure, level of consciousness, and respiratory rate (see Chapter 36). However,
the respiratory rate is particularly important in chest-injured
patients. The oxygen saturation as measured by a pulse
oximeter is very important for monitoring and a baseline
measurement should be obtained in all patients with significant chest injuries. (When recording oxygen saturation, note
the inspired oxygen concentration.)

Signs of injury (e.g. wounds or tenderness) should be
localized. This can usually be done by defining the rib or

intercostal space (by counting down from the manubrio-sternal junction which is at the second intercostal space) and by relating the position to e.g. the anterior axillary line, the midclavicular line, or the costosternal junction. For example:

'stab wound 2 cm long, left 7th ICS, mid axillary line'

or

'Typical seat belt bruising across chest from right clavicle down across sternum. Tender midsternum and right 3,4,5 costal cartilages at costosternal junction'

The examination of the heart and lungs will be done and recorded in the same way as for a medical chest problem and the amount of information recorded will depend on the clinical circumstances.

Examples of notes on chest injury

History:
Fell in shower 7/7 ago, knocked left side of chest
Not been off work, not taken any analgesia
Not SOB, no cough
Came today as pain no better.
PMH: Nil.
O/E:
Looks well
Tender left 6th rib AAL, some pain on springing chest
Chest BS left = right = NAD
P 80, RR normal.
Diagnosis: Minor chest wall injury.

or

History:
In a fight. stabbed in right chest. Brought in by police. refuses to give more details.
Says no pain, not SOB.
O/E:
Looks well, not distressed
Appears alert but unco-operative
P 90, BP 130/85, RR 14, sO$_2$ 95%

Wound 1.5 cm left 6th ICS between MCL & AAL
BS right > left
PN right = left
Trachea central
Ht sounds I & II—normal
JVP not raised.
Abdomen: soft, no tenderness, guarding or rebound normal
bowel sounds.
Diagnosis: ? small left pneumothorax
X-ray:

or

History:
Fell 2/7 ago coming down stairs, tripped and fell down about
5 steps
Landed on right side injured chest. No other injury
Yesterday started to cough—yellow sputum, some specks of
blood
Today more SOB than usual.
PMH:
COAD on ventolin and becotide inhalers
Prednisone 5 mg om
Can usually walk ¼ mile
Smokes 10/day
Nil else.
O/E:
P100, BP 170/95, RR 22, T37.8°C
Tender over a large area of right chest wall in region of ribs
5–10 MAL—PAL
Bony crepitus felt over ? 6th rib
BS left = right = vesicular but scattered wheezes all areas
Heart sounds I & II—NAD
Diagnosis: Chest infection in patient with rib fractures com-
plicating COAD.
X-ray chest:

Major injuries

In a significant chest injury the patient should be managed
and the notes kept in the way suggested in Chapter 36. Any

patient who is short of breath must have the position of the trachea noted as tension pneumothorax is a diagnosis to make and treat clinically before the patient is X-rayed. For example:

History: Stabbed left chest.
O/E: P 140, BP 95/40, RR 35, sO$_2$ (on O$_2$) 80%, GCS 14.
Airway: NAD
Breathing:
Obviously SOB, central cyanosis
Breath sounds decreased on left
Trachea deviated to right.
Diagnosis: Tension pneumothorax.
For: Needle thoracentesis.

NB This is only the first part of the primary survey, much more will need to be recorded during the secondary survey.

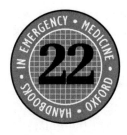

CHAPTER 22

Abdominal injury

History

Mechanism of injury

An accurate history is important as it may not only help in establishing the diagnosis but may assist in the management of the patient. A blow to the abdomen with the force of a kick may cause injury to a solid organ (e.g. spleen), but in these circumstances it can often be treated conservatively. A more severe force such as occurs in a high velocity road accident may injure liver, spleen, or kidney but may also injure a hollow organ. If further investigation reveals intra-abdominal bleeding, a high velocity injury is much more likely to need to be surgically explored.

Current symptoms

In the conscious patient, pain will usually be the major symptom but it can sometimes be difficult to differentiate between pain from the abdominal wall or lower ribs and pain from an injury in the upper abdomen. The presence of shoulder tip pain suggesting diaphragmatic irritation may assist in the diagnosis of an abdominal cause for the pain and so should be asked about but its absence does not exclude such a cause. (Ensure that the patient does not have a shoulder injury to account for pain there!) The presence and type of pain must be sought as the vital signs and initial physical examination of the patient with an abdominal injury may be completely normal and the presence of pain alone will be an indication to admit the patient and probably to investigate them further. If a patient does not present for some hours after an injury, haematuria or vaginal bleeding may need to be asked about.

Past medical history

This should always be established as it may influence the diagnosis and management. Apart from the general points discussed in Chapter 4, diseased organs (e.g. the enlarged spleen or the pre-existing aortic aneurism) or abnormally sited ones (e.g. the transplanted kidney) are more likely to be injured than normal ones. If a patient has had an organ removed in the past there is clearly one less structure to be injured but it may also cause additional problems (e.g. the renal injury in a patient with a solitary kidney).

Examination

As in all patients with significant injuries it is important to record the vital signs.

The examination of the injured abdomen must be meticulous and the results of the examination well recorded. Some injuries may be obvious on admission but others may not and the management of the injured abdomen may depend on the changing physical signs rather than the signs on arrival. The patient should be stripped and the examination of the abdomen should include an examination of the perineum and genitalia.

Marks, and particularly bruises of the abdominal wall, are uncommon and their presence should raise the possibility and even probability of a serious injury. Not only should the presence of all marks and bruises be noted but if there are no marks, in a patient with pain, this should also be noted too.

The abdomen, including the loins, must be palpated and any areas of tenderness identified. As the bruising of lower chest wall injuries may extend into the upper abdominal wall and the fracture haematoma of pelvic fractures may also extend into the abdominal wall, it is important to try to localize the point of maximum tenderness to either the abdomen itself or the the adjacent chest or pelvis. Guarding or rebound tenderness must also be noted and must be assumed to be due to an intra-abdominal cause unless this has been excluded by further investigations.

Bowel sounds must be listened for and the result recorded although the presence of bowel sounds early after the injury does not exclude a significant injury.

A rectal examination must be considered part of the routine examination of the injured abdomen. The presence of blood would indicate a bowel tear and rarely bony fragments from a pelvic fracture may perforate the rectum. The position of the prostate gland should also be noted. In the multiply-injured patient the rectal examination would be done with the patient log-rolled on to their side and combined with an examination of the posterior chest and abdominal walls for wounds, bruises etc., an examination of the spine, and testing for sacral sensation. The anal tone should also be noted on rectal examination as part of the neurological examination. A vaginal examination may, on occasion, also be performed.

In a patient with a pelvic injury, it is essential to exclude a ruptured urethra as this is a contraindication to urethral catheterization. Signs of a urethral injury in a male include blood at the meatus, bruising and swelling of the penis and perineum, and a high prostate on rectal examination. Before any attempt at catheterization in a male with a pelvic injury, the notes should read something like:

'No blood at meatus
No swelling penis
Prostate normal position—for catheterization'

(Perineal bruising is common with a pelvic fracture without urethral injury and by itself would not contraindicate catheterization.)

or (as long as it can be demonstrated elsewhere in the notes that these things have been looked for):

'Catheterization—no contraindications'

An examination of the urine is an essential part of the examination of the abdomen.

Measurement of the abdominal girth not only is valueless but it may be misleading and so should not be done.

Associated injuries

Abdominal injury is common following road accidents and other causes of multiple injuries, and in these circumstances it is particularly associated with chest, pelvic, and lumbar spine injury but it may coexist with any other injury. Following such accidents the patient will need to be examined from head to toe (see Chapter 36). With less severe mechanisms of injury there is still a close association between abdominal and chest injuries and so the chest must be examined in every patient with an abdominal injury (see Chapter 21). This is particularly so with penetrating injuries, as a stab wound anywhere in the upper abdomen or a gunshot wound anywhere in the abdomen has a high possibility of penetrating the chest.

Examples of notes on abdominal injury

History:
Football, went for tackle and fell. Accidently kicked in left posterior chest and loin. Unable to continue game but was able to walk off. Waited 20 mins but pain didn't ease and so came here.
Says moderate pain
Has some pain behind left shoulder
PMH: Appendix age 8, nil else.
Drugs: Nil.
O/E:
P88, BP 120/80, RR 18
Looks well, alert and orientated
Abdo:
Appendix scar, no bruising,
tender LUQ with a little guarding and mild rebound tenderness

Also tender but rather less so in loin and over lower posterior ribs 10–11
Liver, spleen, kidneys not palpable
Normal bowel sounds
Chest:
Not SOB
Breath sounds left = right = normal.
Left shoulder: Not tender, full ROM
Urine: Clear.
Diagnosis: Probable splenic injury.

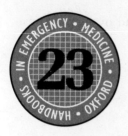

CHAPTER 23

Shoulder injury

That 'X-rays' are not the be all and end all of establishing a diagnosis in traumatized patients is perfectly illustrated in the shoulder where there are several skeletal injuries not shown or easily missed on routine shoulder X-rays but in which correct clinical method will lead to correct X-rays being taken.

History

Most shoulder injuries are caused by a fall on to the out-stretched arm or onto the shoulder itself. If a shoulder injury occurs in a violent muscular contraction, such as occurs in an epileptic fit or an electric shock, there is a high probability that the patient will suffer a posterior dislocation. This injury is easily missed on an antero posterior X-ray and it is important to note the mechanism so that additional views can be taken. Other mechanisms of injury to note include a fall on to the shoulder which may cause a dislocation of the acromioclavicular joint and the acute shoulder pain that occurs during heavy lifting or some similar muscular contraction which may represent a tendinous rupture, usually of the long head of the biceps.

Examination

Look

Many shoulder injuries, including dislocations of the gleno-humeral, acromioclavicular, and sternoclavicular joints, and fractures of the clavicle have characteristic deformities which may be visible and, if a patient presents some days after an injury, bruising may indicate a significant injury. For example, bruising below the level of the deltoid indicating a dislocation of the shoulder or a fracture of the neck of the humerus. Although anterior dislocation of the shoulder usually produces a characteristic deformity, a normal appearance does not exclude this injury especially if the patient is obese. In addition, while inspection of the shoulder should always compare the injured with the uninjured sides, this may miss the rare bilateral shoulder dislocations. It is said that with the patient sitting, inspection of the shoulders from above may reveal posterior bulging in patients with a posterior dislocation.

Feel

Palpation of the shoulder should start by feeling the whole length of the clavicle and the joints at either end not just to localize the point of maximum tenderness but also because deformity may be more easily felt than seen. Injuries of the sternoclavicular joint may be very difficult to visualize on standard X-rays and dislocations and subluxations of the acromioclavicular joint may reduce when the patient lies down. A patient showing clinical signs of an injury here may require stress X-rays for subluxations or dislocations to be adequately demonstrated. The clavicle cannot be X-rayed in two planes at right angles and so an undisplaced fracture of this bone is yet another injury which cannot be excluded on a single AP X-ray. It should not be missed if clinical examination is adequate. Immediately below the clavicle is the coracoid which should be also felt as injuries of this, while rare, may require an axial X-ray to be demonstrated.

The scapula should also be examined for tenderness as fractures may be best demonstrated on 'scapula views' rather than routine shoulder X-rays. Tenderness of the upper humerus probably indicates a fracture at this site and the abnormal position of the anteriorly dislocated humeral head can usually be felt.

Move

The various joints of the shoulder girdle allow the arm to have a very wide range of movement in all three planes. The correct terminology to describe shoulder movements has been the subject of much discussion and confusion. For practical purposes in the injured patient, however, it is only necessary to consider abduction, flexion, and internal and external rotation. Approximate normal ranges of movement are:

- Abduction: 0–180°
- Abduction (glenohumeral joint) 0–80°
- Forward flexion: 0–180°
- Internal rotation (arm at side): 0–90°
- External rotation (arm at side): 0–70°

In the patient with an obvious seriously injured shoulder the examination of movement will be deferred until after X-ray but in other patients, the examination of movement is an essential part of the clinical assessment. The first step is to gently examine rotation of the shoulder. This should not be significantly restricted in injuries of the clavicle and its articulations or in injuries of the scapula. A fixed internal rotation deformity (i.e. the arm is held internally rotated and cannot be put in a neutral position) is highly suggestive of a posterior dislocation of the glenohumeral joint. Abduction of the arm involves a combination of glenohumeral movement until full abduction of this joint has occurred followed by scapula rotation on the chest wall to allow almost 180° of combined abduction. This scapula movement also causes movement at the acromio- and sternoclavicular joints and abduction will be reduced in most shoulder injuries. Decreased abduction is therefore a non-specific sign but abduction should be tested to complete the assessment of shoulder function. It is also necessary to abduct the arm to obtain the axial view required for diagnosing or excluding posterior shoulder dislocations and other injuries. The examining doctor who cannot persuade the patient to abduct the arm to 70° cannot insist that the radiographer tries for an axial view.

In the patient with an acutely injured shoulder it is sufficient to document the range of combined abduction of the arm. However, in the patient with a less acute injury and diminished abduction, it is important to assess how much movement is occurring at the glenohumeral joint and how much is due to movement of the scapula. This is done by placing one hand on the scapula while the shoulder is abducted. The amount of glenohumeral abduction is measured by the angle of the arm at the time the scapula starts to move.

Shoulder function is dependent on the range of movement. Without abduction one cannot comb one's hair and without internal rotation (and extension) a woman is unable fasten her bra behind her back. In the longer-term follow-up of patients it is possible to combine a measurement of range of abduction and internal rotation with a measurement of function by noting (for internal rotation) how far up the back the patient can get their hand (e.g. to buttock, to waist, to T12 or to T6) and (for abduction) how far up they can get their hand (e.g. to nose, to top of head, to back of head).

Alternatively, shoulder movements can be expressed as an approximate percentage of the normal as detected by examination of the other side.

Other tests

Shoulder injuries may be complicated by neurovascular injuries. These are not common except in patients with an inferior dislocation of the shoulder but are well recognized and should be examined for and their presence or absence noted in all appropriate cases. Recognized complications are:

Anterior dislocation: axillary nerve injury
brachial plexus injury (rare)
Inferior dislocation: brachial plexus injury
axillary artery injury
Posterior dislocation of the sternoclavicular joint: pressure on the innominate vessels
Fracture upper humerus: axillary nerve injury
radial nerve injury

Examples of notes on shoulder injury

History:

Known epileptic 20 years. Has fits 2–3 × per year

Fit today normal pattern according to wife. Lasted about 1 minute. Nothing provoked it. Not missed medication.

Somehow injured right shoulder. ? exact mechanism.

No other injury.

Medication: Phenytoin 100 mg tds.

O/E: In pain

No obvious deformity

Generally tender around shoulder joint but no obvious bony tenderness.

ROM: abduction 0–70°0 (but painful ++)

       rotation held in about 50° fixed IR.

Diagnosis: Clinically a posterior dislocation.

X-ray: AP and axial views.

or

History:

Yesterday afternoon

Tripped up a step and fell, put out hand to save herself

? how landed ? on to shoulder ? on to outstretched hand

Left shoulder painful ever since. Couldn't sleep last night.

PMH: . . .

Medication: . . .

O/E:

No deformity

Tender around neck of humerus, nowhere else.

ROM: IR   ¾

     ER   approx. ½

     Abd.   50°

            Diagnosis: ? # neck humerus.

            X-ray: Confirms undisplaced # surgical neck left humerus.

            Radial nerve: power √

            Axillary nerve: sensation √ power √

Non-traumatic shoulder problems

The initial examination of the painful but non-injured shoulder is very similar to that of the injured shoulder but with some additional features.

Look

Deformity;
Muscle wasting especially of deltoid and supraspinatus which may indicate axillary and suprascapular nerve palsies.

Move

The movements to be tested are the same as in the injured shoulder but shoulder abduction should always be separated into glenohumeral and scapulothoracic movements. On abduction, a painful arc should be differentiated from other painful movements and measured e.g.

'Painful arc 60–120°'

Sometimes its absence needs comment. A hand should be placed on the shoulder during abduction and crepitus, if present, should be noted.

Other tests

Rotator cuff disease. Too often all soft tissue shoulder pain is loosely and incorrectly diagnosed as 'frozen shoulder'. This is a specific diagnosis and is one of the less common causes of shoulder pain. The commonest cause of chronic shoulder pain is disease of one or other of the tendons of the rotator cuff or of the subacromial bursa, and by careful examination it is possible to establish an accurate diagnosis. If there is inflammation or a partial tear in a muscle or its tendon, contracting the muscle against resistance will cause pain. Stressing each tendon of the rotator cuff in turn will localize the site of any pain. Pain on resisted abduction indicates a supraspinatus tendonitis, pain on resisted internal rotation indicates subscapularis tendonitis, and pain on resisted external rotation indicates infraspinatus disease.

A painful arc with no pain on resisted movements indicates a painful subacromial bursa. Restriction of active and passive movements in all directions suggests either a synovitis or (more usually) an adhesive capsulitis (frozen shoulder). A diagnosis made in this way is more accurate than localizing soft tissue problems by palpation and will aid the accurate placement and effectiveness of steroid injections.[1]

Winging of the scapula. Sometimes a patient localizes pain to the scapula region or says that there appears to be a lump behind the shoulder. In these circumstances or if examination suggests the scapula is not lying flat against the chest wall, winging of the scapula should be looked for by asking the patient to push their hands against a wall.

Instability. A history of a documented dislocation of the shoulder clearly indicates the possibility of future instability but occasionally patients present with a history suggestive of recurrent subluxation which reduces spontaneously. Stability should be tested with the shoulder in abduction and external rotation.

Examination of the neck. Referred pain from the neck to the shoulder is not uncommon and in a patient with shoulder pain and no abnormality on examination it is essential that the neck is examined. This will include a neurological examination of the upper limb which will detect the occasional brachial plexus problem (especially a Pancoast's tumour) presenting as shoulder pain.

Examples of notes on shoulder examination

O/E:
Tenderness (poorly localized) anterior and point of shoulder
Full ROM but painful arc 60–1000
Pain + on resisted abduction, resisted IR & ER painless.
Diagnosis: Supraspinatus tendonitis

or

O/E:
Shoulder:
No tenderness
Full painless active movements
Resisted movements all painless.
Neck:
No tenderness
Full flexion, lateral flexion and rotation to right Extension
approx. ¾ normal and painful Lateral flexion and rotation
to left approx. ½ normal and both exacerbate shoulder pain.
Power L = R = strong in all groups arms
Sensation L = R = normal
Reflexes L = R = brisk in both arms.
Diagnosis: Pain from cervical spine referred to shoulder.

Reference

1. Hollingworth, G. R., Ellis, R. M., and Hattersley, T. S. (1983).
   Comparison of injection techniques for shoulder pain: results of
   a double blind, randomised study. *British Medical Journal*, **287**,
   1339–41.

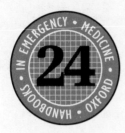

CHAPTER 24

Elbow injury

History

It is important to take an accurate history of the mechanism of injury as there are a number of mechanisms which may give clues to the diagnosis. In one injury in particular the history alone is almost diagnostic. The 'pulled elbow' (subluxation of the proximal radio-ulnar joint) in children is caused by a longditudinal force applied to the forearm. This may occur by the child wanting to go in one direction and the mother pulling in another (hence the name 'temper tantrum elbow') but it is more commonly caused by the father picking the child up by the hands to put it onto his shoulder or to swing it round. It may also be caused by the child holding on to something to prevent a fall, but whatever the cause, the history of a pulling injury to a child's arm followed by the child not using the arm is almost diagnostic of a pulled elbow.

Other mechanisms of injury which may act as pointers are: a fall on the outstretched hand causing a fracture of the radial head or neck; and a fall on to the point of the elbow which may cause a fracture of the olecranon or of a condyle. The extra energy of a fall from a height (e.g. a climbing frame) is usually necessary for a child to have a supracondylar fracture and a forced rotation of the forearm may cause the rare dislocation of the radial head.

Examination

Look

Three injuries cause deformity at the elbow. The commonest are a supracondylar fracture of the humerus and a dislocation of the elbow. Less common is a dislocation of the radial head either as an isolated injury or, more commonly, as part of a Monteggia fracture dislocation involving a fracture of the ulna. Other things which should be looked for are swellings, either of the joint itself (i.e. an effusion) or of the olecranon bursa.

Feel

If the elbow is deformed, palpation of the relationship between the olecranon and the condyles will differentiate between a supracondylar fracture and a dislocation. In the former injury the normal equilateral triangular relationship between the olecranon and the two condyles is preserved but in a dislocation it is disrupted.

In the less severe injury palpation is useful to confirm any swelling and to localize any tenderness. The bony points to be palpated are the two condyles, the olecranon as noted above and the radial head. The soft tissues which can be easily identified are the biceps, triceps, and brachioradialis tendons and the ulna nerve running behind the medial epicondyle. It is important to localize and record the most tender area. If initial X-rays do not show an injury, one may need to do further views. For example, if the X-ray request states:

'Fell on outstretched hand, tender radial head',

and the initial X-ray shows radiological evidence of an effusion but no bony injury the radiographer will probably do additional oblique X-rays of the radial head and/or radial head capitellum views. This additional help will not be obtained if one has not localized the tender area and the X-ray request states merely:

'Fell, injured elbow'.

Move

When moving the elbow the range of movement in both elbow and radio-ulnar joints should be noted. Normal elbow movement is from 0–150° of flexion (but some patients can hyperextend their elbows up to 15° and their range of movement would be expressed as −15 to 150°. Normal supination is from 0–90° and pronation from 0–80°.

An elbow effusion, which is almost inevitable with any acute intracapsular fracture will cause loss of movement at the elbow joint especially extension. The injured elbow which has a full range of movement probably does not need to be X-rayed. Pain on forearm rotation may indicate a radial head fracture but severe loss of forearm rotation is usually caused by either subluxation or dislocation of the radial head or by fractures more distally in the forearm. The typical history of the child with a pulled elbow combined with loss of supination confirms the diagnosis of a pulled elbow and one can proceed to manipulation without an X-ray.

Other tests

The significantly displaced elbow injury, either a supra-condylar fracture or a dislocation, may have an associated injury of either the brachial artery or of one of the nerves which crosses the elbow (most commonly the median nerve). It is important that circulation and nerve function are examined distal to every significant elbow injury and adequate notes made. The examination for vascular and nerve injuries are described in Chapters 34 and 35.

Two rare injuries of the elbow are closed avulsions of the biceps and the triceps tendons. They are much less common than the closed rupture of the long head of the biceps tendon which occurs at the shoulder but they are important to recognize as they need surgical repair. If they are suspected from the history of the patient feeling something 'go' in the elbow while the muscles are contracted and from the localization of the tenderness to the tendons, the integrity of the tendons should be tested. On resisted elbow flexion the biceps tendon normally stands out but if the tendon has ruptured or been avulsed this will not be felt and flexion will be weak.

If triceps avulsion needs to be excluded, the patient should be asked to stand with the shoulder abducted to 90° and the forearm dangling and then to extend their arm against gravity. They will be unable to do so if the tendon is not intact.

Associated injuries

A common mechanism of injury to the elbow is a fall on to the outstretched hand. In the elbow this typically causes fractures of the radial head but the same mechanism may also cause wrist injuries e.g. a Colles' or a scaphoid fracture. Injuries of the forearm and wrist may also cause restriction of or pain on forearm rotation and it is important to examine the forearm and wrist as part of the elbow examination. If this examination is normal consider referred pain and examine the shoulder.

X-rays

An effusion is almost inevitable following an intra-articular fracture. This is not always easy to detect clinically but radiological evidence of an effusion (i.e. the 'fat pad sign') is a good indicator of a fracture even if it cannot be seen on the initial X-rays. When writing down the interpretation of the X-rays one should note the presence or absence of an effusion in addition to details of any bony injury.

Examples of notes on elbow injury

History:
Fell 4 feet off climbing frame on to grass. ? how exactly he landed but screamed immediately. Only apparent injury is to right elbow.
Has walked since.
PMH: Fit healthy child. No significant problems.
O/E:
In pain, crying + +
Obvious deformity right elbow with bruising
Normal relationship between olecranon and condyles

Radial pulse normal, hand warm, normal colour and capillary return

Passive wrist movements normal

Difficult to test nerves but appears to have normal sensation all areas of hand. Won't co-operate with testing muscles

No other obvious injuries. Impossible to assess tenderness but full passive movement wrist, hand.

Provisional diagnosis: Supracondylar fracture.

X-ray:

or

History:

This a.m. slipped on wet kitchen floor, fell on to outstretched left hand. Injured left elbow.

PMH: On ibuprofen for OA knees, nil else

O/E:

Left elbow slightly swollen with effusion

Tender radial head

ROM: 20–90° full rotation but painful

Wrist not tender, full ROM

Clinically fracture radial head

X-ray: NBI but positive fat pad sign.

or

History:

Weightlifting yesterday and felt something 'go' in left elbow followed by pain. Couldn't continue. This morning bruised and more painful

O/E:

Bruising antecubital fossa

Tender around bruised area

Full passive ROM, elbow and forearm rotation

Decreased power in elbow flexion, biceps tendon not palpable.

Diagnosis: Closed biceps avulsion.

Non-traumatic elbow problems

History

The commonest symptom in the elbow is pain and the most usual causes are 'tennis' and 'golfers' elbow. While both may be due to over-use in sport, most are caused by work or 'do it yourself' over-use injuries, especially tasks which involve much pronation and supination of the forearm e.g. using a screwdriver.

Mechanical symptoms in the elbow (e.g. locking) are rare but almost always indicate a loose body within the joint either from osteochondritis dissicans or from osteoarthritis.

Late ulna nerve palsies may follow malunion of supracondylar fractures and must be looked for in appropriate cases.

Examination

The examination of the uninjured but painful elbow is the same as that of the injured elbow but there are additional tests for specific problems. If a biceps or triceps tendonitis is suspected then pain on resisted elbow flexion and extension respectively will help to confirm this. 'Tennis elbow' is caused by a lesion at the common extensor origin on the lateral epicondyle and so resisted movements of the muscles having their origin here (finger and wrist extensors and supinator) will be painful. 'Golfer's elbow' is a similar condition occurring at the common flexor origin and can be tested for by pain on resisted wrist flexion and pronation.

Example of notes on non-traumatic elbow pain

History:
Pain right elbow 3/12. Gradual onset. No trauma.
Pain worse when grips things—affecting his work—carpenter.
Getting worse. Eased when had 2 weeks holiday but then returned as soon as he went back to work.
Has had no treatment for this.
O/E:
Tender + one spot lateral epicondyle
Full ROM: (a bit painful last 10° of extension) full rotation
Pain on resisted wrist extension and pain ++ on resisted supination.
Diagnosis: Tennis elbow.

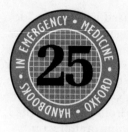

CHAPTER 25

Forearm and wrist injuries

Forearm injury

History

There are a variety of ways in which the forearm can be injured, including falling or becoming caught in machinery, but the history of a blow with a heavy stick or similar object to the ulna aspect of the forearm (e.g. when the forearm has been raised for protection against assault) should suggest the possibility of an isolated fracture of the shaft of the ulna (nightstick fracture).

Physical examination

The only specific point to make about the examination of the injured forearm, apart from to follow the usual routine of: look; feel; move; circulation; and nerve supply distal to any fracture, is that one needs to examine elbow, wrist, and radio-ulna joints. If it seems that a patient has an isolated fracture of one of the forearm bones it is important to exclude a dislocation of either the superior or inferior radio-ulnar joints.

Significant blunt trauma to the forearm may, even in the absence of a fracture, cause a compartment syndrome (see Chapter 34).

Examples of notes on forearm injury

History:
Breezeblock fell about 1 foot on to forearm this a.m. at work. Continued to work but after about ½ hour became more painful and so came to hospital.
TT booster 3 years ago.
O/E:
Superficial abrasion c. 6 × 5 cm dorsum of forearm. A bit swollen and tender
Full painless ROM elbow, wrist, forearm rotation
Grip strong but causes pains in extensors upper forearm
Radial pulse, sensation normal.
Diagnosis: Bruising and abrasion forearm, no evidence compartment syndrome.

or

History:
Assaulted, attacked with hockey stick, put up left arm to protect himself and hit on ulna aspect arm.
Now painful ++ can't use arm
No other injuries.
O/E:
Brusing lower ⅓ ulna
Tender most of subcutaneous border of ulna, maximally at junction of upper ¾ and lower ¼
Full painless elbow movements, wrist about 30° flexion and extension only
Pronation about 20° no supination at all
ulna deviation causes pain +.
Clinically: # distal ulna.
X-ray radius and ulna:

Wrist injury

History

As for all parts of the body the mechanism of injury may suggest the diagnosis and so must be recorded.

A fall on to the outstretched hand will commonly cause a greenstick fracture of the radius in children, a fractured scaphoid in young adults, and a Colles' fracture in older adults (especially those with osteoporosis). It should not be forgotten that a goalkeeper who puts up his hand to stop a ball and injures his wrist in the process has suffered the same mechanism of injury and is also at risk of a scaphoid fracture. A fall on the outstretched hand may also cause a minor chip fracture of the triquetrum, either alone or in association of one of the other injuries.

By contrast, a forced hyperextension injury without a blow may cause a dislocation of the lunate and a starting handle kick-back (now seen in people starting machinery on construction sites) classically causes a fracture either of the radial styloid or of the scaphoid. (If the kick-back is to the thumb rather than to the wrist, a Bennett's fracture dislocation is the common result.)

The 'Colles' fracture' occurring in young people as a result of a high velocity injury (e.g. a road accident) is a different and more serious injury than that which occurs in osteoporotic bones following a fall and is much more likely to incur soft tissue complications such as vascular and nerve injuries.

A direct blow to the hypothenar eminence (e.g. a golfer whose club hits the ground rather than the ball) may cause a fracture of the underlying hook of the hamate. This is a rare injury but as this fracture is not visible on standard wrist X-rays an accurately recorded history of the mechanism may prevent this fracture from being overlooked.

Apart from pointing towards a diagnosis, an accurately recorded history may also be useful as a means of excluding a diagnosis. For example, a patient whose injury was caused by a direct blow to the wrist (e.g. with a hammer), is unlikely to have a fractured scaphoid.

The past medical history may be very important in interpreting the X-rays and in deciding treatment. Scaphoid fractures are frequently missed initially and lead to long-standing scaphoid non-union with or without secondary degenerative disease. When a patient re-injures his wrist and the X-ray shows non-union one needs to be able to recognize this as long-standing. The patient may know the diagnosis but even if not he will probably be able to relate that the wrist is always 'weak'. Colles' fractures do not develop non-union but very commonly heal with marked residual angulation and radial shortening. If such a patient re-injures their wrist it will look worse than the severity of the acute injury suggests. Colles' fractures tend to occur in the elderly who have many pre-existing medical problems, and it is necessary to take these into consideration when planning treatment. There may be no point in manipulating a fracture in a wrist which is never used because of a hemiplegia. In a patient with serious cardiac disease it is necessary to weigh the benefits of a marginally improved position of the fracture against the risks of anaesthesia for manipulating it.

Examination

Look

The 'dinner fork' deformity of a Colles' fracture is usually obvious but occasionally a Smith's fracture may have associated swelling on the dorsum of the wrist which obscures the underlying anterior angulation. Similar deformities are seen in children with fractures of the distal radius or the epiphysis.

Scaphoid waist fractures are usually associated with swelling in the anatomical 'snuff box' and its absence makes a fracture unlikely even if there is snuff box tenderness.

Feel

The distal radius and ulna and the whole wrist should be palpated. Minor degrees of deformity may be more easily felt than seen. The point(s) of maximum tenderness should be accurately identified and noted. This is particularly important on the radial side of the wrist where the radial styloid, the scaphoid in the anatomical snuffbox and the base of the first metacarpal lie very close together. It is very common for patients with disease at the base of the first metacarpal, de Quervain's syndrome and fractures of the radial styloid to be falsely diagnosed as having a clinical scaphoid fracture due (in part) to poor localization of tenderness.

The anatomical snuff box should be routinely palpated and such is the medicolegal importance of the fractured scaphoid that it is useful to routinely note the result. If the snuff box is tender then additional signs of a scaphoid fracture should be sought such as tenderness over the scaphoid tubercle, swelling, pain on telescoping the thumb, and reduced wrist movements.

Other bony landmarks which are easily identified are the ulna styloid, the distal radio-ulna joint and, anteriorly, the pisiform. On the dorsum of the wrist the carpal bones are easily felt but it is difficult to identify each one although a knowledge of anatomy should assist in trying to identify the tender area (e.g. the hamate articulating with the base of the fifth metacarpal or the triquetrum on the ulna side of the wrist in the proximal carpal row). On the palmar aspect of the wrist the scaphoid tubercle and the pisiform have been mentioned. The hook of the hamate is also on the palmar aspect and while it cannot be felt it is situated in the hypothenar eminence distal to the pisiform and tenderness here should alert one to an injury of the bone.

Move

The wrist movements with normal ranges are:

flexion	75°
extension (dorsiflexion)	70°
radial deviation	20°
ulnar deviation	30°
pronation	70°
supination	85°

These can all be easily measured although it is not necessary to routinely measure radial and ulna deviation in the acutely injured wrist.

Other tests

Median nerve compression commonly occurs in association with severely displaced fractures of the distal radius and dislocations of the lunate and it is also a not uncommon complication of a simple Colles' fracture and so should be routinely looked for in these patients.

Associated injuries

As noted in Chapter 24, there may be an association between wrist injuries and fractures of the radial head, both of which may be caused by a fall on the outstretched hand. The elbow should be examined in all such patients.

Examples of notes on wrist injury

History: Fall on outstretched hand.
O/E:
No deformity, swelling or bruising
Maximally tender ASB and to a lesser extent over radial styloid. Not tender scaphoid tubercle. No pain on telescoping thumb
Full ROM, slight pain on full flexion. Full rotation
Elbow NAD.
Probable sprain but in view of ASB tenderness—X-ray.

or

No deformity. Swelling ASB.
Tender ++ ASB and anterior of scaphoid.
ROM:
extension about ⅓ normal. pain ++
flexion about ⅔.
Elbow NAD.
Diagnosis: clinically a # scaphoid.
X-ray:

or

Dinner fork deformity with bruising ++
Tender + distal radius and ulna styloid. Not tender ASB
Sensation in all fingers normal
Elbow NAD.
Diagnosis: clinically a Colles' #.
X-ray:

Forearm and wrist wounds

Every laceration of the forearm and wrist, no matter how superficial, should be assumed to have divided important structures until proved otherwise. Many tendon or nerve injuries are missed because it is thought unnecessary to examine function in so superficial a wound. The structures examined will depend on the site of the wound but it is better to do a fuller examination than necessary than miss something. When the wound is sutured it should be explored and details of this exploration noted.

Examples of notes on wrist lacerations

History:
Went to push open a door and hand went through a glass panel. First aider bandaged it and called ambulance.
Last tetanus toxoid > 10 years ago.
PMH: Nil significant.
O/E:
4 cm deep transverse laceration palmar aspect wrist.
FDP √√√√   FPL √
FDS divided to index and middle
FCU and FCR appear intact
Ulna n Ab Dig Min √
          sensation √
Median n decreased sensation middle and index fingers, thumb appears normal
Ab Poll Br difficult to test because of pain.
Diagnosis: Partial median nerve injury and division FDS to index and middle fingers.
X-ray to exclude glass FB: No FB seen.
Refer hand surgeon.

Non-traumatic wrist and forearm problems

The examination of the patient with non-traumatic problems in the wrist is essentially as described for the injured wrist but there are some additional tests which should be done in certain circumstances.

Apart from unrecognized injury the most common causes of wrist pain in A&E practice are tenosynovitis and similar problems. Tenosynovitis crepitans is caused by over-use and presents with pain and a characteristic palpable crepitus when the wrist is moved. In any patient with soft tissue pain in the lower forearm and certainly in any patient diagnosed as 'tenosynovitis' or '? tenosynovitis' this should be looked for and its presence or absence recorded.

De Quervain's syndrome (tenovaginitis of the tendons of abductor pollicis longus and extensor pollicis brevis) is another common cause of wrist or thumb pain. The patient presents with pain in the area of the radial styloid (but as noted above, poor localization on clinical examination may confuse pain here for anatomical snuff box tenderness). Despite the pain being in the radial styloid, wrist movements are relatively painless and the pain is exacerbated by thumb movement. There may be a lump and crepitus but the diagnostic test is that forced thumb flexion and resisted thumb abduction are painful. Pain from the first carpometacarpal joint can also be confused with wrist pain and so thumb movements must be examined and noted in anyone with pain on the radial side of the wrist and tests for de Quervain's syndrome must be done frequently.

Example of notes

History:
Pain right (dominant) wrist 2/12. No trauma. No over-use. Made worse by using hand. Nothing eases it. Getting worse. GP gave a crepe bandage and topical ibuprofen—no help. No pain at night.
PMH: Nil, no wrist injuries or joint problems.
O/E:
Tender radial styloid, nowhere else. Small lump over styloid
Full painless ROM wrist and forearm rotation. No crepitus
Thumb movements full but uncomfortable

Pain + on forced thumb flexion and resisted thumb extension.

Diagnosis: de Quervain's syndrome.

Carpal tunnel syndrome

This is a common cause of wrist, forearm, and hand pain presenting to A&E. Early in the disease the patient may have symptoms on waking and after use but there may be no signs on examination. The history is therefore all important and should contain details of:

• Possible causes (e.g. trauma, pregnancy),
• Timing of symptoms especially pain at night and paraesthesiae on waking
• Which fingers are affected?

Examination. The neurological examination of a patient with a suspected carpal syndrome is the same as that of a patient with a median nerve injury at the wrist (see p. 129). In addition, the patient's symptoms may be reproduced by tapping the anterior surface of the wrist over the carpal tunnel (Tinel test). If the symptoms are in any way atypical, the neck should be examined and a full neurological examination of the arms performed.

In addition to the neurological examination one should look at the patient's face and ask oneself the question 'Does the patient look as if they have got myxoedema or acromegaly?' as these uncommon predisposing conditions are so easily overlooked.

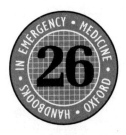

CHAPTER 26

Hand injury

Key points in hand injury

- The fingers must be named and not numbered.
- Note whether the patient is left or right handed.

Naming of fingers

The digits should always be named[1] and never numbered, to avoid the confusion caused by the index finger being the second digit but the first finger and the errors which have resulted from this. The digits are called:

- Thumb
- Index finger
- Middle finger
- Ring finger
- Little finger

The middle finger can also be described as the long finger to avoid any confusion in the similar sound of little and middle. The metacarpals are normally numbered 1 to 5 but they too can be described in relation to their digit (e.g. the first meta-carpal can be described as the thumb metacarpal, the second as the index metacarpal etc.) The web spaces are usually numbered 1 to 4 but can be described as e.g. 'Web between index and middle'.

History

While it is important in any upper limb injury to know whether the dominant or non-dominant side is injured, it is even more important in the hand. It is also important to know, not only a patients' occupation, but also their hobbies and interests and where this is of relevance it should be noted. This will influence the advice, prognosis, and reassurance given to patients and in patients with serious injuries it may directly affect the patients management by enabling a surgeon to decide on the correct treatment when there is perhaps a choice between an operation to restore strength and one to allow dexterity.

The history of a hand injury is important. A direct blow to a digit may cause a contusion or a fracture but a hyperextension or similar injury may cause a fracture but is more likely to cause an injury at a joint. A laceration of the finger tip caused by a sharp object must be distinguished from the 'burst' laceration caused by a crush injury. The latter may well harbour an underlying fracture but will swell considerably and should not be sutured initially.

Another factor of particular importance in the hand is function. It is important to ask the patient what they can and cannot do. If the patient needs prompting one can ask specifically about work, home life, and recreational activities. It is a disaster to operate on a hand which has some deformity but functions perfectly and to end up with a normal-looking hand that does not work.

Past medical history

Not only is the hand frequently injured but it is also the site of congenital deformities (e.g. curved little finger) and other problems (e.g. Dupuytren's contracture) which patients may not have recognized and so may blame on an acute injury. Previous problems may need to be asked about, and as problems are frequently bilateral, examination of the other hand may be useful.

Examination

Wounds

The examination and note keeping for wounds has been described earlier (Chapter 14). However, it is useful to emphasize the need to examine tendon and nerve function distal to every wound. The description of wounds on the hand may be difficult and so diagrams are essential and will convey much more information than the written word (e.g. Fig. 26.1). Most A&E departments have a selection of rubber stamps and the proforma of the British Society for Surgery of the Hand is particularly useful (Fig. 26.2)

If a patient complains of interference with hand function it is usually possible to test this in the consulting room. For example grip strength can be simply tested by asking the patient to grip a hand and fine tasks can be observed by asking the patient to do up their buttons or shoelaces or pick

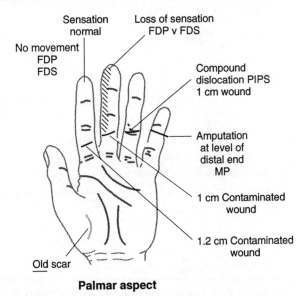

Palmar aspect

Fig. 26.1 • A diagram is sometimes more useful than a thousand words.

Hand injury chart

Hospital

LEFT
dominant hand: left/right

Number
Name
Address

Occupation

Date of birth
G.P.

Age

M/F

History

Date of injury..
Time of injury..am/pm
Details of injury

Where		How caused		Type of wound (circle as appropriate)	
home	☐	knife	☐	open/closed	
work	☐	glass	☐	tidy/untidy	
RTA	☐	machinery	☐	cut/crush	
sport	☐	burns	☐	clean/dirty	
other		explosive	☐	skin loss	yes/no
		other		amputation	yes/no

Accident ☐   Assault ☐   Self inflicted ☐

avulsion   yes/no

Examination by Dr/Mr...

Indicate clearly: lacerations, skin loss, amputations
sensory loss, bone injuries, retained foreign body

on ....

X-Ray   yes/no
Photograph   yes/no

Ulnar border cf .... finger   Radial border of .... finger   Details ....

Tendon Injuries (circle those divided)				Nerve Injuries (circle those divided)	Circulation	
Thumb	APL/EPB	FPL	EPL	median	Normal	yes/no
Index	FDS	FDP	ED/EI	ulnar	Details	
Middle	FDS	FDP	ED	radial		
Ring	FDS	FDP	ED	digital (specify)		
Little	FDS	FDP	ED			

Fig. 26.2 • Proforma for hand injury. (© British Society for Surgery of the Hand, and reproduced with kind permission.)

up paper clips one by one. Note can be made of how easily and quickly they do the tasks, which parts of the hand they use, and which parts they avoid using.

Thumb injuries

Feel

On palpating the thumb it is important to localize the point of maximum tenderness and, as noted above, it is particularly important to differentiate between tenderness at the first carpometacarpal joint and scaphoid tenderness.

Move

The thumb has three joints. Movements of the trapezium—first metacarpal joint—are difficult to measure but adduction, abduction, rotation, and a small amount of flexion (about 15°) occur here. The ranges of flexion at the other joints are:

Interphalangeal joint	0–80°
First metacarpophalangeal joint	0–50°

If a joint is injured, its movement should be measured but as a test of function it may be useful to measure the composite movement of opposition. This is the movement in which the thumb moves across to touch the tip of the little finger and further flexion brings the tip of the thumb to the base of the little finger. A measure of opposition is the distance between the tip of the thumb and either the tip of the little finger or the base of the the little finger at full stretch.

Ligamentous sprains at the first metacarpophalangeal joint are very common but it is essential not to miss a complete rupture of the ulna collateral ligament at this joint. This is a very disabling injury but is easily repaired if diagnosed early. In all injuries of this joint its stability should be tested (although it can wait until after the X-ray if one suspects a fracture at this site).

Examples of notes on hand injury

History:
Right handed.

Last night fell on ski slope. wearing gloves. Right thumb got caught in mesh. Couldn't continue. Went home. Still painful this a.m. despite aspirin.

O/E:

Right 1st MCPJ swollen + and tender especially over ulna side.

ROM 0–20°0 (other side 0–40°0)

Stability left = right but pain on stressing ulna collat lig

Full painless ROM IP & 1st CMCJ

Diagnosis: sprain ulna collat lig Right 1st MCPJ.

or

History:

3/52 ago. cricket. fell injured right (dominant) thumb ? hyperextension injury.

Saw GP told clinically NBI and given crepe bandage.

Since then, no better. Can't work (plumber) as can't grip things

O/E:

Fading bruise thenar eminence. No swelling

tender 1st MCPJ but maximally tender base 1st MC.

1st MCPJ stable.

Whole thumb very stiff (tip of thumb 4 cm from base little finger).

Provisional diagnosis: exclude missed fracture or dislocation.

X-ray:

Metacarpal and finger injuries

Finger movements

Fingers move at the metacarpophalangeal, the proximal, and the distal interphalangeal (IP) joints. The average movements are:

Metacarpophalangeal joint	flexion	90°
	extension	45°
Proximal IP joint	flexion	100°
Distal IP joint	flexion	80°

The range of movement for an injured joint must be recorded but for a measure of hand function, one can look at the total flexion of the finger. When making a fist the finger tips can normally touch the proximal palmar crease. Any loss of total finger movement can be measured by the distance of the finger tip from the proximal palmar crease on making a fist. The distance between the finger tip and the distal palmar crease can be used as a measurement of composite movement at the proximal and distal interphalangeal joints.

It is sometimes convenient to look at all the fingers together and to assume that, because a patient can fully extend all the fingers and appears to make a full fist, they have a full range of movement of all the metacarpophalangeal and interphalangeal joints. If they can make a tight fist then this is true but it is easy to overlook the one distal interphalangeal joint that has not flexed.

The importance of examining tendon and nerve function distal to any wound has been stressed. However, closed tendon injuries also occur. Mallet deformity is well recognized but rupture of the central slip of the extensor tendon is easily overlooked and closed flexor tendon rupture may be missed as it is not often considered.

Closed metacarpal and finger fractures
Particular points to note

Fractures of the metacarpals, proximal and middle phalanges, and any associated displacement or angular deformity will usually be seen easily on an X-ray. This will not demonstrate rotatory deformity which can only be detected clinically and must be looked for and corrected in any fracture of these bones. A note should be made that this has been done. Rotatory deformity may not be obvious if the patient's hand is flat but on flexion, the fingers normally move in parallel with the tips pointing to the thenar eminence. If there is a rotatory deformity, the affected finger will tend to curl under or over the adjacent fingers. If the patient cannot flex the fingers, the finger tips should be viewed end on, when the affected finger nail will not be parallel to the rest.

Proximal interphalangeal joint injuries

Particular points to note

In all proximal interphalangeal joint sprains, it is important to test the stability of the collateral ligaments and consider the possibility of an extensor tendon central slip rupture.

Examples of notes on hand injury

History:
Right handed
Last night punched a wall in anger, injured right hand.
O/E:
Bruising and swelling 5th MCP joint
Joint held in 20° flexion
Tender distal 5th MC
ROM active 20–90°, passively can be got straight but no hyperextension
No rotatory deformity
Clinically # neck 5th MC.
X-ray:

or

History:
Right handed. injured right index finger
3/52 ago went to catch a cricket ball, bent finger back,
Didn't seek help at time, thought it would get better.
Since then pain easier but still painful if he knocks it and still very stiff (NB keen guitarist—finds it difficult to play).
O/E:
PIPJ swollen and tender especially radially.
ROM 20–80° only. finger about 2 cm from palm on making a fist
Stable
MCPJ and DIPJ normal.

or

History:
This p.m., playing rugby went to tackle someone and right

ring finger got bent back. now painful and doesn't move properly.

PMH: # right scaphoid 2 years ago nil else.

O/E:

Slightly swollen and tender around DIPJ

PIPJ normal

Full passive movement DIPJ but appears to have no active flexion at all

Extensor tendon normal.

Diagnosis: Closed rupture FDP.

X-ray to exclude an avulsion #.

Reference

1. Medical Defence Union and Royal College of Nursing of the United Kingdom (1978). Joint Memorandum. *Safeguards against wrong operations*. Medical Defence Union, London.

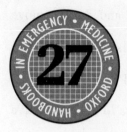

CHAPTER 27

Lower limb injury

Key points in lower limb injury
- Examine the gait.

History

It is important to establish whether a patient has walked since the accident. This may be obvious (e.g. if the patient walks into the consulting room) but a patient with a knee or hip injury will often have been asked to undress and lie on a couch before being seen by the doctor and it may be necessary to ask specifically. A patient who has walked normally or run since they injured themselves is unlikely to have a serious injury, but the ability to weight bear does not always exclude a significant fracture.

Examination

The importance of examining and making a note of a patient's ability to weight bear and walk was made in Chapter 6, and certainly no patient with a lower limb or back problem should be allowed home without a comment on their gait recorded in the notes. A patient with a seemingly minor injury who will not weight bear must be re-examined and almost certainly needs to be X-rayed.

Even if a patient says they are unable to weight bear it is

still important to try to confirm this by getting the patient to his or her feet once a significant injury has been excluded either clinically or by X-ray. Many patients say they are unable to weight bear when they mean that they limp and others who cannot walk when they enter the A&E department are able to walk out once they have been reassured by a normal X-ray.

When making notes about the gait, the type of gait should be described if possible e.g.

'Walks with knee held absolutely straight'
'Walks on tip toes, will not put heel to ground'
'Walks confidently with one stick'

or, in patients with pre-existing disease:

'hemiplegic gait' 'Parkinsonian gait' etc.

It is not enough to say that a person limps but one should give some indication as to how severe it is. Grading a limp in the notes could be as simple as:

'limp'
'limp +'
'limp ++'
'limp +++'

The individual doctor who writes this will know what is meant but it is more informative to describe the severity of a limp e.g.

'negligible limp'
'minimal limp'
'moderate limp'
'severe limp'
'hardly able to weight bear'
'refuses to put foot to ground—hops'

In a more chronic problem and if there is any doubt about whether there is a limp, it can be very imformative to look at the patient's shoes as uneven wear on the soles will confirm that there is a problem and may give some indication of the type of problem.

Hip injuries
Mechanism of injury

In the elderly it is important to determine that the 'fall' causing a hip injury was a genuine fall and not the result of a 'blackout' or similar medical problem.

If a fracture has been caused by minimal trauma (especially in the relatively young) this should be noted as the underlying cause (most commonly osteoporosis) may need investigation and treatment.

Mechanisms causing particular injuries include:

1. The knee hitting the dashboard in a road traffic accident causing a posterior dislocation of the hip in addition to a knee injury.
2. The side impact on a car door causing a central dislocation of the hip.
3. The young person who gets acute pain around the hip at the height of athletic exertion is likely to have an avulsion fracture.

Other features in the history

Most hip injuries, and especially fractures of the neck of the femur and single pubic rami fractures, occur in elderly patients who are likely to have other medical problems and disabilities. Past medical problems (e.g. osteoporosis) are frequently an underlying cause of the hip injury. Dislocation of a total hip replacement can occur, and it is important to enquire about the past medical history including previous surgery. Details of this may take up more of the A&E record card than details of the hip injury itself. Note should also be made of the patient's social circumstances and their pre-injury mobility. If these were poor, admission may be required following a hip injury even if there is no fracture. If the patient requires admission nurses, social workers, and occupational and physiotherapists will write many reports but a line on the A&E card saying e.g.

'Lives alone in a bungalow, daughter visits twice a week, no home help, uses a stick when she goes shopping'

is sufficient at this stage.

Examination

Look

The position of the leg should be observed. A patient with a fractured neck of femur typically appears to have a shortened and externally rotated leg. Children with a significant slipped upper femoral epiphysis also hold their leg in external rotation while the patient with a posterior dislocation of the hip holds it flexed, adducted, and internally rotated.

Move

As with all injured patients one should use common sense before moving an injured hip. The examination of a patient with a very painful injury sustained a short time earlier will be different from that of a patient who has been walking on a painful hip for two days. An initial approach to testing movements is to gently rotate the hip by internally and externally rotating the foot with the leg extended. If this is acutely painful stop, but if it is not painful test hip movements as described below.

Apparent flexion and extension of the hip can be caused by rotation of the pelvis caused in turn by movement of the lumbar spine. A patient with a fixed flexion deformity of the hip can lie on a bed with their legs flat if they lie with an increased lordosis of their lumbar spine. Hip flexion should be examined with the other hip flexed so as to abolish any lumbar lordosis and reveal any fixed flexion deformity.

Hip extension is measured with the patient lying prone but there is usually little need to measure this in A&E practice.

When measuring abduction and adduction the pelvis should be fixed with the examiner's other hand to ensure that movement is occurring at the hip and not the pelvis.

Internal and external rotation of the hip are easiest to measure with the hip flexed but if this is painful they can be tested with the leg extended. These can be important movements to measure as the earliest sign of a slipped upper femoral epiphysis is loss of internal rotation.

Average hip movements are:

flexion	110–120°
extension	30°
abduction	50°
adduction	30°
internal rotation (hip flexed)	45°
external rotation (hip flexed)	45°

Special tests

The sciatic nerve lies behind the hip joint and may be injured in patients with a posterior dislocation of the hip. It should always be examined in such patients.

Displaced fractures of the pubic ramus may be associated with a bladder injury and the appearance of the urine should be noted in all cases.

Examples of notes on hip injuries

History:
Tripped over carpet this a.m., fell on to left hip
Pain ++ no other injuries
Couldn't get up, ambulance called, not walked since
Lives with husband, independant.
PMH:
Right total hip replacement 2 years ago
Ca breast 15 years ago, no recurrences
Asthma (moderately severe but never been in hospital with it)
TB as a child.
Drugs:
coproxamol (for OA knees)
predisolone 5 mg om
bendrofluazide 5 mg om
salbutamol inhaler
becotide inhaler.
O/E:
obese, left leg held shortened and externally rotated
vaguely tender around hip, difficult to localize pain
comfortable at rest but any movements of hip cause pain +.

Diagnosis: # neck femur.
X-ray to confirm:

or

RTA patient
O/E:
In pain ++.
right leg held flexed, internally rotated and adducted bruising over patella, no obvious effusion knee but difficult to examine as kept flexed because of hip injury hip movements not tested because of pain.
Sciatic nerve sensation √ ankle movements √.
Clinically: posterior dislocation hip, difficult to exclude knee injury.
X-ray:
right hip
right knee.

or

Child 14
History:
fell off roller skates yesterday onto right hip
not able to continue to skate but limped home
pain in hip and front of thigh
pain worse today.
PMH 'clicking hip' as baby, settled with no treatment, nil else
O/E:
no deformity,
vague redness and some bruising over gtr trochanter
tender over bruised area and to lesser extent over pubis

ROM	Right	Left
flexion	90°	120°
abduction	right	= left
adduction	right	= left but painful on right
IR	30°	50°
ER	45°	45°

Gait walks with foot turned out, marked limp.
Provisional diagnosis: probable soft tissue injury but need to exclude slipped upper femoral epiphysis.
X-ray right hip AP and lateral:

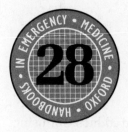

CHAPTER 28

Knee injury

Mechanism of injury

Many of the important injuries of the knee are of the soft tissues and not visible on plain X-rays. Most diagnoses can be made clinically but even for those diagnoses requiring more specialized or invasive procedures (e.g. Magnetic resonance imaging or arthroscopy), good clinical skills are needed to select the patients who require further investigation.

The first clue towards the diagnosis is to understand the mechanism of injury. A direct blow to the knee itself may cause a fracture or a contusion but it will not cause a sprain or a meniscal injury. A force that tends to move the tibia in relation to the femur is likely to cause a ligamentous injury whereas for a meniscal tear one requires a twisting injury while weight-bearing. The knee that suddenly collapses during exertion might suggest a rupture of the extensor mechanism, whereas recurrent giving way points towards a mechanical problem within the knee joint or some instability possibly caused by weak quadriceps muscles. A dislocated patella which has reduced spontaneously can only be diagnosed by obtaining a history that the patella moved laterally and then returned to its normal position.

What happened next

A patient who sustains a knee injury and is able to finish his game of football is highly unlikely to have a significant injury.

If the patient has an effusion it is essential to know how quickly this accumulated. An effusion which forms within half an hour is a haemarthrosis which suggests either an intra-articular fracture or a tear of a vascular structure such as a ligament. If the X-ray is normal, the commonest cause of a haemarthrosis is a tear of the anterior cruciate ligament with or without other injuries. An effusion which does not form for several hours suggests a serous effusion or traumatic synovitis possibly due to a meniscal tear.

Past medical history

Many knee injuries occur in footballers and other sportsmen who will have had previous injuries, some of which may not have been fully diagnosed or from which they may not have fully recovered. Typical problems are meniscal tears, recurrent dislocation of the patella, instability from an anterior cruciate rupture, and functional instability caused by weak quadriceps muscles. Patients may also have other knee problems such as osteoarthritis or osteochondritis dissecans.

It is essential to ask about previous knee problems in anybody with an acute knee injury and rather than concentrating on the presenting knee injury, it is sometimes more useful to ask questions about the first time they ever injured their knee. If a patient does have previous knee problems, one should ask specifically about locking, catching, and giving way which would suggest a mechanical cause such as a meniscal tear or a loose body.

Examination
Look

The stability of the knee depends to a large extent on the strength of the quadriceps and the examination of the knee must include these muscles. Trousers must be removed and not just rolled up, and both thighs should be exposed to allow comparison between the two sides. Wasting of the quadriceps on one side is usually obvious. This can occur within days of an injury. If found immediately after an injury, it is an indication of some previous knee problem or injury from which the patient has not fully recovered and it is likely that the quadriceps wasting itself played some role in the aetiology of the injury. For an acute injury, the state of the quadriceps need only be described in the notes if it is abnormal but for chronic problems it should always be described on the record card. If it is necessary to measure the degree of quadriceps wasting e.g. for medicolegal purposes, to convince a patient that there really is a problem or to act as a baseline before referring a patient for physiotherapy this can be documented by measuring the thigh circumference at a set distance above, say, the upper pole of the patella. (This is not a particularly accurate measurement and need not be done as a routine.)

This can be recorded as e.g.

'Circumference 20 cm above upper pole patella:

Right	Left
54 cm	51.5 cm'

The knee is the easiest joint in which to observe an effusion. If an effusion is visible its presence can be confirmed by palpation. This will also differentiate an effusion from swelling in the prepatellar bursa or periarticular bruising. (This is also important in non-traumatic problems as it is not rare for a septic prepatellar bursitis to be initially mistaken for a septic arthritis.) When the presence of an effusion is documented in the notes there should be some estimate of the size (e.g. minimal, small, moderate or large) and for a large effusion it should be noted whether or not the effusion is tense.

The absence of an effusion shortly after the injury means that an intra-articular fracture or cruciate tear is unlikely. Occasionally a capsular tear in association with a collateral ligament rupture may allow an effusion can escape into the surrounding tissues. An ecchymosis below the medial or lateral joint lines may point towards this injury.

Feel

Palpation of the extended knee is usually easiest for confirming the presence of an effusion and for feeling the patella but the ligaments and joint lines are easiest felt with the knee flexed. The following parts should be identified:

- medial and lateral femoral condyles
- medial and lateral joint lines
- medial and lateral tibial plateaus
- head of the fibula
- patella, patella ligament, tibial tuberosity
- soft tissues to either side of the patella
- tendons behind the knee

As with almost every other injury it is important to identify which bone or soft tissue structure is the point of maximum tenderness. For example, if a patient has pain on the medial side of the knee one may suspect a medial collateral ligament sprain or a medial meniscal tear but if tenderness is localized to the medial femoral condyle, then the pain can be assumed to be from the origin of the ligament and not from the meniscus.

Swellings around the knee should be identified (e.g. Baker's cyst, semimembranosus cyst) and occasionally loose bodies in the knee joint can be felt.

Move

As with any other joint, the range of movement of an injured knee should be recorded (the average range is 135° of flexion with up to 10° of hyperextension) and retropatellar crepitus should be noted. However,if the patient is unable to fully straighten the knee, one should record the feeling at the 'end point' when one tries to straighten the knee. If the limitation to extension is caused by pain and an effusion (the usual cause) there will be a 'spongy' end feel. If there is a mechanical block due to a loose body there will be a solid end feel. A mechanical block due to a meniscus tear will give a 'springy' end point.

Knee flexion in the supine patient requires that the hip flexes too. If a patient has hip problems such that flexion is too painful to allow the knee to bend up, then the patient can be turned on to their side allowing knee flexion without moving the hip.

Stability

In any knee injury the integrity of the cruciate and collateral ligaments should be tested and compared to the other side. Any instability or pain on stressing the ligaments should be noted.

To test the medial collateral ligament, one hand is placed on the lateral side of the knee joint as a fulcrum and the other holds the ankle and tries to abduct the leg and 'open up' the medial side of the joint. If the ligament is ruptured, there will be an abnormal ammount of 'give' or 'opening up'. Instability when the knee is straight only occurs if there is laxity of the cruciates in addition to the medial ligament and so stability should be tested with the knee in 20–30° of flexion. The lateral collateral ligament is tested similarly.

To test for cruciate laxity, the knee should be flexed to 90°. The examiner sits on the examination trolley and stabilizes the foot with his own body. He then grasps the upper tibia and jerks it backwards and forwards. Excessive forward movement from a neutral position indicates an anterior cruciate tear and excessive backwards movement, a posterior cruciate injury (Drawer test). The acutely injured knee may not bend to 90° but the examiner with large hands may be able to grasp the lower femur with one hand and the upper tibia with the other and, with the knee in a few degrees of flexion, try to move the tibia forwards and backwards on the femur. Excessive movement indicates a cruciate rupture (Lachman test).

Circulation and nerve supply distal to an injury

The popliteal artery is at risk of injury in any patient with a dislocation of the knee or a supracondylar fracture of the femur and the circulation should be tested in all these patients. These are severe injuries, with major soft tissue damage, and so the nerve supply to the foot must also be tested.

The lateral popliteal nerve runs on the postero-lateral side of the knee and round the neck of the fibula and is vulnerable to injury in patients with a fractured neck of fibula and rupture of the lateral collateral ligament of the knee.

Other tests to diagnose specific injuries

Testing for integrity of the extensor mechanism. Ruptures of the quadriceps tendon and patella ligament are commonly missed. The former is associated with a normal X-ray and it is entirely a clinical diagnosis. The X-ray of the latter will show a patella which is too high and this may not be obvious to an inexperienced observer. If either is suspected (history of the knee giving way, an injury to the anterior part of the knee and—in patients with a quadriceps tendon rupture—a palpable gap between the tendon and the upper pole of the patella), the integrity of the extensor mechanism must be examined. The first test is to ask the patient to do a straight leg raise. If this can be done, the extensor mechanism is intact. However, many patients with an acutely painful knee are unable to straight leg raise because of pain and so the patient should be sat on the edge of the bed and asked to extend the knee against gravity. An inability to do this (in the context of an acute injury) confirms the diagnosis. In patients with a quadriceps tendon rupture, the gap above the upper pole of the patella will get bigger as the quadriceps contract.

Apprehension test for dislocating patella. Dislocation of the patella is often a recurrent problem. A patient with the patella still dislocated can be diagnosed from the end of the bed. However, the patella usually reduces spontaneously and it may be difficult to diagnose unless a clear history is obtained that the patella moved laterally and then returned. Recurrent dislocation may present as repeated giving way of the knee. If the diagnosis is suspected one should do the 'apprehension test'. The patella is pushed laterally as if to dislocate it and the patient, sensing that it is about to dislocate, suddenly contracts the quadriceps to prevent this from happening. This is a positive apprehension test.

McMurray test for meniscus tear. This is usually too painful to do on the acutely injured knee but it should be done on the less acute knee injury if one suspects the diagnosis. To test the medial meniscus, the knee is fully flexed and the foot is externally rotated. With a hand over the knee, the leg is abducted and then the knee is smoothly extended. Palpable 'clicks' and 'clunks' indicate a meniscal tear. For the lateral meniscus, the test is repeated with the foot internally rotated.

Examination of the hip

Patients who complain of pain in the knee following an injury and in whom there is little abnormal to find on examination, should have their hip examined. It is by no means rare for hip problems to present with thigh or knee pain. This typically occurs in patients with a slipped upper femoral epiphysis but can also occur in other conditions such as femoral neck fractures.

Treatment

As with all injuries the treatment prescribed and advice given should be documented as described in Chapter 10. However, as implied above, quadriceps wasting is very common and a major cause of continuing problems following a knee injury. It is largely preventable and so notes for a knee injury must contain a line such as:

'Quads exercises demonstrated and advised' *or*
'Quads advice sheet given'

as part of the advice given.

Examples of notes on knee injury

History:
Football yesterday. went for a tackle and somehow injured right knee. ? exact mechanism
Unable to continue playing but could walk on it
Swelled up overnight.
PMH: Nil significant, no previous knee injuries/problems
O/E:
moderate effusion
ROM 10–100°

tender medial femoral condyle
stable but tender ++ on stressing medial collat. lig.
moderate limp
McMurray not done
Diagnosis: sprain medial collat. lig.

or

History:
1 hr ago, tripped on a loose stone, fell onto gravel path
landed on left patella. Unable to weight bear and so called
ambulance
Tet tox course 7 years ago.
PMH:
mild angina takes GTN (< 1 in 2/52)
nil else
O/E:
Very superficial 3 cm laceration transverse over patella
Large tense effusion
Tender everywhere but especially over patella
ROM: very reluctant to move at all
Stability: collats stable in extension but not possible to test
cruciates as can't bend knee
Provisional diagnosis: # patella (wound superficial and so
not compound).
X-ray:

or

History:
Today jogging through woods, right foot stumbled over a tree
root. Put weight on left leg to save himself but left knee 'gave
way' and he fell to ground. Found he could walk if he kept
knee straight.
PMH: No previous knee problems
O/E:
Knee swollen but no obvious effusion
Slightly tender around upper patella
Full ROM
Stable
Gait: walks with knee held straight, if knee bends then can't
support weight

Can't SLR, can't extend knee against gravity, palpable gap above upper pole patella
Diagnosis: rupture quads tendon.

or

History:
twisted right knee playing football 1/52 ago
swelled up by following day
better than it was but not right
2 previous similar problems in past year.
first time twisted it in a tackle, couldn't continue,
swelled up, couldn't play for 2/12
no locking, catching, giving way between injuries.
PMH: arthroscopy for ? medial meniscus left knee 3 years ago
(under Mr Sawbones)
O/E:
Quads wasting
Small effusion
Well-healed scar over patella (laceration as a child)
Tender anteromedial joint line
ROM: 5°—full flexion
Stability: lat lig seems slightly lax but left = right
Minor limp
McMurray painful but no click felt.
Provisional diagnosis: Probable medial meniscus tear.

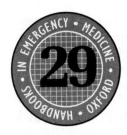

CHAPTER 29

Leg and calf injuries

Key points in leg and calf injuries
- If there is ANY possibility of an Achilles tendon injury, Simmond's test is essential

---

Examination

The tibia runs subcutaneously throughout its whole length and tenderness is easily localized. The examining doctor must, however, not neglect the fibula as although isolated fractures of this are much less significant, they are easily and frequently overlooked in e.g. the footballer who has been kicked.

The patient who develops acute pain in the calf while exerting themselves (typically running for a bus or playing squash) is likely to have one of three injuries. Rupture of the medial head of gastrocnemius and a tear in the musculo-tendinous junction of the muscle can be distinguished by localizing the point of maximum tenderness. It is important the correct history is obtained as, when they present late, these injuries may be misdiagnosed as deep vein thrombosis. The calf is easiest to examine with the patient either lying prone or kneeling on a chair. The third injury which presents with the same history is a rupture of the Achilles tendon. This may be suspected by tenderness over the tendon rather than the muscle or musculotendinous junction and a gap in the tendon may be palpable. If there is any possibility of this injury, Simmonds' test must be performed. The patient lies prone with their feet over the edge of the trolley and the calf is squeezed. If the Achilles tendon is intact, the foot will plantar flex but if the tendon is ruptured, the foot remains still.

The lateral popliteal nerve may be injured in association with fractures of the upper fibula and so should be examined in all patients with such injuries.

The lower leg is the commonest site for compartment syndromes in the absence of bony injury. These are discussed in Chapter 34.

Examples of notes on leg and calf injuries

History:
Football. Went in for tackle ? what happened but severe pain right lower leg. Unable to move. Ambulance called.
Splinted and brought here. Ambulance men found abnormal movement when splint applied.
PMH:
right tibia and fibula 12/12 ago in M/C accident. Treated in POP for 15/52. Discharged from # clinic 4/12 ago.
Nil else
O/E:
In pain. Right leg in splint (not removed)
No obvious deformity
Very tender junction of middle and lower 1/3 with swelling.
Knee not tender and no effusion
Ankle not tender
Sensation in foot—normal, can move toes
Foot normal colour, warm, dorsalis pedis pulse present
Gait: not examined.
Diagnosis: # right tibia and fibula.
Morphine 12 mg given by slow titration caused pain to ease.
X-ray tibia and fibula:

or

History:
Yesterday afternoon football, kicked on outer side right leg. Continued to play for 15 mins but then became more painful and so came off.
O/E:
No bruising. Tender mid fibula. Not tender tibia.
Full ROM knee and ankle. Moderate limp.
Diagnosis: exclude # fibula.
X-ray tibia and fibula: Undisplaced # midshaft fibula.
Lateral popliteal nerve: good power ankle dorsiflexion (but painful)

or

History:
Yesterday running for bus, sudden severe pain in back of left calf and 'felt something go'. Difficulty in walking afterwards but much more painful today and can hardly walk.
O/E:
Lower calf swollen and bruised + +. Tender musculotendinous junction of gastrocnemius. Achilles tendon NOT tender.
Achilles tendon intact (Simmond's test)
Foot held in plantar flexion, can get foot to a right angle but dorsiflexion causes pain + +.
Gait: Can hardly walk at all.
Diagnosis: Tear gastrocnemius.

or

History:
Playing squash. Sudden pain lower left calf 'thought my opponent had hit me with his raquet.' Couldn't continue.
PMH: Steroid injection for ? Achilles tendinitis 6/52 ago.
O/E:
Tender Achilles tendon with palpable gap.
Limp
Simmonds' test: ruptured Achilles tendon.

Non-traumatic problems
Pain in the calf

One of the most serious causes of pain in the calf is deep vein thrombosis and the notes should make it clear that this has been considered. Also, the possibility of deep vein thrombosii and its complication of pulmonary embolus excluded. For example, in a patient with a probable ruptured Baker's cyst the notes should include something like:

'*History*:
No VVs, no PMH or FH of DVT/PE, not on oral contraceptive
No chest pain, no shortness of breath
O/E:
Tender calf +, no ankle oedema, no VVs
Moderate limp
Not tender femoral vein, chest clear
No evidence DVT'

However, if there is significant doubt, a venogram will be required.

Pain in shin

There are many causes of shin pain but the majority of patients with this symptom in A&E are athletes and the differential diagnosis will include a stress fracture, shin splints, chronic strain of the muscular attatchments to bone, and tenosynovitis. Recent exertion and training schedules should be noted and on examination crepitus of tenosynovitis should be looked for and resisted movements of the ankles and toes examined to see if they reproduce the pain. For example:

History:
Running to try to get fit to join Royal Marines.
Recently increased mileage from 3 to 7 miles per day.
Pain in Left shin started last week after 1 mile. Getting worse, now has to stop after ½ mile.
PMH: . . . .

O/E:
Tender medial border tibia middle ⅓. Appears not to be bony tenderness
No crepitus
Pain on resisted ankle dorsiflexion
Full painless ROM knee & ankle
Gait: minor limp.
Assessment: probable shin splints but need to exclude stress #.

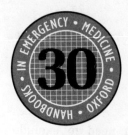

CHAPTER 30

Ankle injury

Keypoints in ankle injury

- Fractures of the fifth metatarsal and calcaneum are commonly misdiagnosed as sprained ankles and so palpation of these areas is an essential part of the examination of the ankle.

History

The commonest mechanism of injury at the ankle is an inversion injury and it is easy to fall into the trap of assuming that every ankle injury has been caused in this way. However, there are other mechanisms of injury which occur at this site and there are two injuries which would be missed much less frequently if a proper history was taken. Ruptured Achilles tendon has been noted above under the heading of calf injuries (Chapter 28) but it may also be misdiagnosed as a sprained ankle by the careless. The other injury commonly missed is the fractured calcaneum. The clue to this injury is that it is usually caused by a fall directly on to the heel.

Other mechanisms of injury worthy of note include the forced dorsiflexion injury (typically occurring in the road accident when the pedal on which the driver's foot is resting is shunted backwards) which may cause an injury to the talus and (also in road accidents), the foot which tangles with the pedals possibly causing midtarsal and tarso-metatarsal dislocations.

A history of recurrent inversion injuries of the ankle suggests the possibility of instability due to a ruptured lateral ligament. It is more commonly due to functional instability due to damage to proprioceptive nerve fibres and to muscle weakness from a previous injury but this history will normally mean that a stress X-ray should be obtained.

Examination

There have been several studies to establish the clinical features that differentiate a sprained ankle from a fracture following an inversion injury. These are:

- *Age* (the older the patient, the more likely a fracture).
- *The ability to weight bear* (which makes a significant fracture less likely).
- *The point of maximum tenderness* (patients with a fracture of the lateral malleolus will be tender over the bone whereas maximum tenderness over the anterior or inferior parts of the lateral ligament makes a significant fracture highly unlikely).
- *Swelling* (this is a less sensitive indicator but fractures in the absense of swelling are unlikely).

It would be difficult to justify a decision to X-ray or not to X-ray without this information, and these details must recorded in every case.

Fractures of the calcaneum and ruptures of the Achilles tendon have already been noted as commonly missed injuries but another injury which may be overlooked is the fracture of the base of the fifth metatarsal. This too is caused by an inversion injury of the ankle and is commonly associated with a sprained ankle (less commonly with an ankle fracture) and will be missed if not specifically looked for. Palpation of these three areas should become a routine part of the examination of the ankle. Diastasis of the lower tibio-fibular joint in the absence of a lateral malleolar fracture will be associated with a fracture of the mid part or upper fibula and this too may be missed.

Move

Ankle movements are flexion (plantar flexion) and extension (dorsiflexion) but at the same time as looking at movements of the ankle joint, inversion and eversion should be examined. These movements occur at the subtalar and midtarsal joints. Subtalar movements can be examined by holding the heel and measuring passive inversion and eversion in relation to the tibia. Midtarsal movement is examined by holding the heel still and observing inversion and eversion of the foot in relation to the stationary heel.

Although it is not easy to be accurate, these can all be measured in degrees. Average ranges are:

Ankle   flexion 48°
           extension 18°
Subtalar   inversion 5°
           eversion 5°
Midtarsal inversion 33°
           eversion 18°

Special tests

As in all parts of the body it is important to examine the circulation and nerve supply distal to a displaced fracture.

In patients with wrist and hand lacerations it is accepted that one should examine for tendon and nerve injury in every patient, no matter how superficial the wound appears. Lacerations of the ankle and foot are much less common than in the upper limb but similarly one should test any tendon or nerve which could have been injured.

Associated injuries

A fall on to the heels from a height commonly causes bilateral fractures of the calcaneum and may also cause a crush fracture of a vertebra. In any patient with a calcaneal fracture, it is necessary to ensure that this is not a bilateral injury and also to examine and, if necessary, X-ray the lumbar spine.

Examples of notes on ankle injury

History:
Today jumped off a 4 ft wall onto concrete path.
Landed flat on heels. Severe pain left heel. Can't weight bear on left foot.
No back pain
O/E:
Hopped in on right foot being supported by wife
Left ankle:
Bruising + heel and tender ++
Not tender med or lat malleoli but tender below both malleoli
Full ROM ankle joint but pain ++ on subtalar movement
Not tender TA, 5th MT or forefoot
Right ankle:
No tenderness anywhere
Full ROM ankle/subtalar/midtarsal joints.
Lumbar spine: no tenderness, ROM not examined.
Clinically: fracture left calcaneum.
X-ray left ankle with calcaneal views: confirms crush # calcaneum, involves subtalar joint

or

History:
Walking in town this a.m., tripped over uneven pavement, inversion injury right ankle
Walked home and sat down but now ankle swollen up.
O/E:
Some swelling around lateral malleolus
Slightly tender lat. mall. but maximally tender anterior talo-fibular lig
Slightly reduced ROM
Walks well but minor limp
No tenderness 5th MT, calcaneum, Achilles tendon.
Diagnosis: sprain right ankle, no indication for X-ray.

or

History:
Yesterday evening coming down ladder, missed last rung and twisted left ankle.

Limped last night but pain kept him awake all night and this a.m. can't weight bear

Went to see GP who sent him here—see letter

PMH: Ca bladder—4 years ago due a check cystoscopy next month.

O/E:

Ankle swollen around both malleoli.

Tender all around ankle but especially over lateral malleolus ROM about ½. Not tender calcaneum, 5th MT, Achilles tendon

Severe limp.

Clinically: lateral malleolus.

X-ray:

or

History:

Taking a pane of glass out of a window, dropped it causing a laceration right ankle.

Applied a dressing and came straight here.

Tet Tox booster 2 years ago.

O/E:

3 cm clean incised wound transverse across anterior of right ankle joint.

Tib ant √ EHL √ extensor dig √√√

Sensation present in all toes

Full ROM ankle, normal gait

X-ray to exclude glass FB:

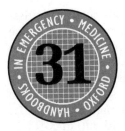

CHAPTER 31

Forefoot injury

Naming of toes

As with the fingers (see Chapter 26), it is important that, in patients with toe injuries (or other toe problems), the toe is correctly identified to avoid any confusion. The present recommendation[1] is that they are called:

1st toe (or big toe or hallux)
2nd toe
3rd toe
4th toe
5th toe (or little toe)

Other nomenclatures have been described including one based on the nursery rhyme 'This little piggy goes to market. . . .'[2] but this will be incomprehensible to those unfamiliar with English nursery rhymes. If names are used, the big, little, and middle toes are easily identifiable and the other two can be named after the equivalent fingers (i.e. the index and ring toes).[3] Whereas the sides of a finger are described as radial and ulna, the sides of a toe are best described as medial and lateral.

History

It is sometimes argued, because the management of a fractured toe is little different from the management of a bruised toe, that toe X-rays are unnecessary for the management of an injury. This ignores the fact that dislocations occur and missing a dislocated toe because of a failure to X-ray might cause long-term problems. The mechanism gives the first clue to the underlying injury. A patient who has dropped a brick on to a toe is likely to have either a contusion or a relatively undisplaced fracture. In such patients it is unlikely that the result of an X-ray will change the management significantly. A decision to treat a patient clinically without an X-ray in such cases is perfectly acceptable. On the other hand a patient who has stubbed their toe may have a soft tissue injury, a fracture (which may be displaced) or a dislocation and while a history of a stubbed toe, by itself, is certainly not an indication for an X-ray, it does influence the diagnostic process and therefore the investigations performed.

Other ways of injuring the foot include an inversion injury of the ankle, causing a fracture of the base of the 5th metatarsal (as described in Chapter 30) and the severe crush injury of the foot which typically but not exclusively occurs in a road accident when a driver's foot is crushed under the pedals. This may cause a tarso-metatarsal dislocation which may be overlooked in the presence of other injuries particularly as the X-ray abnormalities may be subtle.

Past medical history

Peripheral vascular disease, diabetes mellitus, and to a lesser extent, other causes of peripheral neuropathy are of particular importance in patients with disorders of the foot. In foot injuries they may delay healing and be a cause of complications. If discovered on taking the history or examining the patient, they should be emphasized in the notes and the notes of many non-traumatic foot problems should not be considered complete without mention of the state of the foot pulses and documentation of the blood sugar.

Examination

The examination of the foot follows the same pattern as described for other parts of the body. Movements of the big toe are easily measured. An average range of movement is:

1st metatarso-phalangeal joint flexion   45°
                                 extension 70°
Interphalangeal joint   flexion   90°

However, denenerative disease of the first metatarso-phalangeal joint is very common (its presence should, of course, be noted) and so movements should be compared to the other side. Movements of the joints of the other toes should be examined as a full range of movement will exclude a dislocation or a recent intra-articular fracture but it is usually not helpful to try to measure them.

Examples of notes on foot injury

History:
Got out of bed this am, walking barefoot and stubbed little toe on doorpost
Says toe is bent and can't get shoe on.
O/E:
Wearing sandals walking on heel
Hallux valgus with overriding of 2nd toe
Little toe bruised and appears deviated laterally
Tender over whole toe
Provisional diagnosis: ? dislocation, ? fracture.
X-ray: fracture proximal phalanx with displacement laterally.

or

History:
Building a wall yesterday, dropped concrete slab on left big toe (no safety boots)
Painful but continued to work though last night kept him awake with throbbing pain.
O/E:
TP swollen, subungal haematoma
full ROM 1st MTPJ, IPJ ROM about ⅔ compared to right
Limp (walking on heel)
Diagnosis: Subungal haematoma, clinically # TP not involving IPJ
X-ray not needed.

Management: Trephine.
Trephining Dr . . . . Red-hot paperclip method, much blood released with much relief of pain.

or

History: Training for marathon, running 25 miles per week on roads
5/7 pain in right foot came on after running—no injury
Not too bad at rest or on gentle walking but can't run
Not helped by ice packs
PMH: Aches and pains in knees and shins from running but nil else.
O/E:
No deformity, bruising, swelling
Tender distal part of 2nd MT and to a lesser extent 3rd MT
Full ROM ankle/subtalar/midtarsal/toes
Minor limp.
Provisional diagnosis: Probable stress fracture 2nd MT.
X-ray:

or

History:
Ingrowing right big toe nail on and off 2 years
Nail removed by GP 18/12 and 6/12 ago
Painful this time for 3/52—not responded to antibiotics from GP ? what.
PMH: Nil.
O/E:
IGTN right lig toe laterally (says never had problems medially).
Not infected
Refer chiropodist for ? lateral wedge excision and phenol ablation.

References

1. Medical Defence Union and Royal College of Nursing. (1978). Joint memorandum. *Safeguards against wrong operations*. Medical Defence Union, London.

2. Heyes, F.L.P. (1992). On the naming of toes—porcine nomenclature. *Journal of the Medical Defence Union*, **8**, 94.

3. Constant, C.R. (1993). On the naming of toes (letter) *Journal of the Medical Defence Union*, **9**, 24.

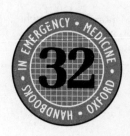

CHAPTER 32

Child limping or unable to weight bear

Key points in limping child injuries

- The child who is unable to bear weight must be examined from hip to toe.

The small child who falls over and refuses to walk without any signs of a major limb injury is a common problem. As the child may be unable to say where the pain is and tenderness may be difficult to localize especially if they are crying, he or she must be examined from the toes to the hip even if the site of injury appears to be in one area. Common injuries causing this problem are greenstick fractures of the first metatarsal, spiral and greenstick fractures of the tibia and, less commonly, greenstick fractures of the femur.

The child who is limping following an injury must be examined similarly but it is less likely there is a fracture of a long bone if the child is walking.

There are many causes of a small child presenting to A&E with an acute onset of limp or refusal to weight bear without any history of trauma. The commonest are:

Unrecognized trauma (including non accidental injury).
Perthes' disease.

172

Irritable hip.
Osteochondritis of the navicular.
Osteomyelitis.

These children must also be fully examined from toe to hip and if no abnormality is found, the back should be examined as discitis and other back problems may also present in this way.

Examples of notes for child refusing to weight bear

History:
Playing in garden, climbed on to dustbin and fell off.
? how he landed.
Now won't put right foot to ground. No other injuries.
O/E:
Won't put foot to ground
No tenderness even to firm palpation toes to hip
Full ROM toes/foot/ankle/knee/hip
X-ray whole right leg:

or

History:
Fell off swing, landed on right side.
Cried immediately, now won't walk on right leg
Parents seem to think it is the ankle which is painful.
O/E:
Puts toes to ground but won't put weight on foot
Foot a bit swollen on dorsum
Difficult to localize tenderness as crying but dislikes being touched there more than anywhere else.
Ankle movement and inversion/eversion full but ? painful
Full ROM knee and hip.
Exclude a # in foot or ankle.
X-ray foot and ankle. If that is normal, X-ray femur and tibia and
fibula.

PART 4

Other injuries

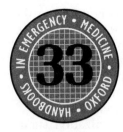

CHAPTER 33

Burns

Key points in burns
- **The only accurate way to calculate the burn area is to use a Lund and Browder chart.**

History

The time that the burn occurred is very important and must be recorded as fluid replacement is calculated from the time of the burn and not from the time of arrival at hospital.

The depth of a burn will depend on the temperature of the burning object and the duration of exposure. Therefore the mechanism of burning should be recorded. A burn from molten metal will almost always be of full thickness whereas a scald caused by a cup of tea will usually be partial thickness or deep dermal. A full thickness burn may be even caused by hot tap water if contact has been prolonged (e.g. if an elderly patient gets into a hot bath and cannot get out). In electrical burns the voltage should be discovered as while almost all electrical burns are full thickness, high voltage burns will cause deeper muscle and nerve injury. Patients with chemical burns sometimes assume that because they have been burnt, the chemical involved must be an acid whereas alkaline burns may frequently be more serious. It is important to identify the chemical as accurately as possible as systemic absorption may occur or there may be specific treatments for the burn. Any treatment already given should be noted.

A very important complication of burns is injury to the respiratory tract caused either by direct thermal injury or smoke inhalation. Physical examination will give many clues to this (see later) but a history of prolonged exposure in a smoke filled room, shortness of breath or coughing up soot particles may raise the suspicion of such an injury and these issues should be explored in appropriate cases.

Burns are wounds and so tetanus immunization status should be recorded.

Examination

The essential information to record for a burn is the same as that required for any wound i.e. location, size, and depth. The depth of a burn immediately after the injury is determined from its appearance and on whether the area maintains its sensitivity to a pin prick. It should not be described as first, second, or third degree as these terms mean different things to different people. One should only describe a burn according to the actual pathology i.e.

- erythema
- partial thickness
- full thickness
- mixed
  or even
- indeterminate

The description of a burn as being of partial thickness or deep is an interpretation and so describe what you see, e.g.

'Burn upper third of dorsum of right forearm 4 × 3 cm, brown, dry, leathery—typical of a full thickness burn'

or

'Partial thickness scald left shoulder and outer aspect of upper arm with blistering'

In a deep burn (e.g. an electrical burn) one should examine underlying structures such as tendons or nerves to exclude involvement of them in the burn.

CHART FOR ESTIMATING SEVERITY OF BURN WOUND

NAME________ WARD________ NUMBER________ DATE________

AGE________ ADMISSION WEIGHT________

LUND AND BROWDER CHARTS

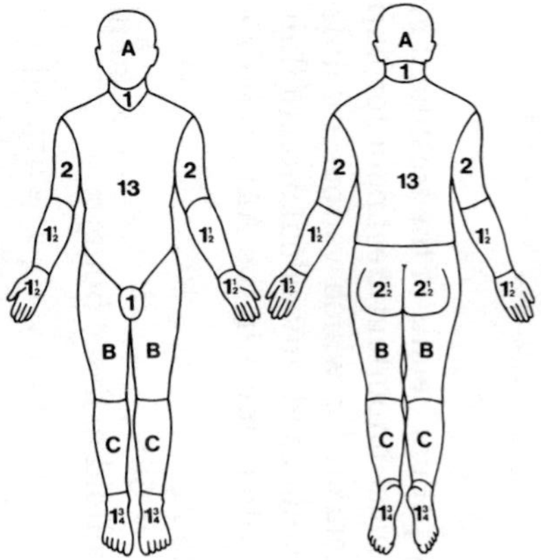

IGNORE
SIMPLE ERYTHEMA

Partial thickness loss (PTL)

Full thickness loss (FTL)

REGION	% PTL	% FTL
HEAD		
NECK		
ANT.TRUNK		
POST.TRUNK		
RIGHT ARM		
LEFT ARM		
BUTTOCKS		
GENITALIA		
RIGHT LEG		
LEFT LEG		
TOTAL BURN		

RELATIVE PERCENTAGE OF BODY SURFACE AREA AFFECTED BY GROWTH

AREA	AGE 0	1	5	10	15	ADULT
A=½ OF HEAD	9½	8½	6½	5½	4½	3½
B=½ OF ONE THIGH	2¾	3¼	4	4½	4½	4¾
C=½ OF ONE LEG	2½	2½	2¾	3	3¼	3½

Smith+Nephew

For further supplies of this pad or of Flamazine* Cream for the prevention and treatment of infection in burns contact Romford (0708) 349333 or your Smith & Nephew Pharmaceutical representative.

*Trade mark

TRANSFER INFORMATION CHART

Contact your Regional Burn Centre early for advice.

TIME OF INCIDENT:

TIME OF ARRIVAL:

HOW ACCIDENT HAPPENED

CLOTHING WORN AT TIME

FIRST AID GIVEN

HOW LONG FOR?

I.V. CANNULA SIZE

SITE OF INSERTION

CATHETER PASSED YES/NO

CATHETER SIZE:

URINE OUTPUT: ml

Time measured:

ANALGESIA/ANTI-EMETICS

AMOUNT	ROUTE	TIME

TETANUS TOXOID (please tick)

UP TO DATE ☐ GIVEN ☐

Transfer form designed with the help of the staff of the McIndoe Burns Centre, East Grinstead, England.

† Available from Smith & Nephew Pharmaceuticals Ltd

SMOKE INHALATION SUSPECTED? YES / NO

SOOT IN THROAT/NOSE YES / NO

HOARSE VOICE YES / NO

INTUBATION REQUIRED YES / NO

SIZE OF TUBE:

BLOOD GASES:
(if taken)

FLUID REQUIREMENT CALCULATION

(see also "Burns a Plan of Action" wallchart)†

WEIGHT OF PATIENT: Kg

ESTIMATED BURN AREA: %BSA

$\frac{\text{WT OF PT} \times \text{\% OF BURN}}{2}$ = Total colloid infusion over four hours

= ml per period

FLUID REGIME – FIRST 4 HOURS FROM INJURY

HOUR	FLUID	AMOUNT
1		
2		
3		
4		

COMMENTS:

Fig. 33.1 • Chart for documenting the extent of burns.

The size of small burns can be expressed in the same way as other wounds e.g.

'partial thickness burn on dorsum of right hand 3 × 2 cm'

However, the size of larger partial and full thickness burns is expressed in terms of the percentage of the total body surface area which the burn covers. Note that this calculation should exclude any erythema. The area is best calculated on a Lund and Browder chart and the chart should form part of the notes. Figure 31.1 shows a proforma for the documentation of burns in the A&E department which is distributed by a pharmaceutical company—it consists of a Lund and Browder chart overprinted with other essential items of the history and examination. This chart may also be used for documenting the exact location of the burn but it may not be sufficient for detailed drawings of the extent of burns to the hand and face when more detailed charts should be used.

In appropriate cases evidence of inhalational injury should be looked for and recorded. Clues to such injury from the physical examination include hoarseness or stridor, burns to the mucosa of the nose or mouth, singeing of the hairs of the nostril, soot particles in the nose, oropharynx or sputum, and wheezing.

Treatment

As with any patient details of the treatment given should be noted. The most important treatment for burns is adequate fluid replacement for which various formulae exist. Whatever the formula used, any calculation of fluid requirements should be written down in the A&E records e.g.

'weight = 65 kg
area of burn = 30%
$$\text{Volume of colloid in first 4 hours} = \frac{65 \times 30}{2} \text{ ml}$$
$$= 975 \text{ ml}$$
$$= 1 \text{ l (approx,)}'$$

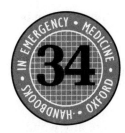

CHAPTER 34

Vascular injury

Key points in vascular injury

- The presence of a pulse does not exclude a more proximal arterial injury.
- Any wound overlying an artery must be assumed to have injured it until proved otherwise.
- In any patient with severe limb pain consider a compartment syndrome.

The circulation distal to any displaced fracture or dislocation should always be examined and noted. The obvious thing to record is the presence of the peripheral pulses but unfortunately this does not reliably exclude an arterial injury. It is possible to have a palpable pulse distal to a complete arterial division because of the collateral circulation. It is important therefore that other tests are employed. The circulation to the skin can be assessed by looking at the skin colour, feeling its temperature, and assessing the capillary return. The adequacy of skin blood supply can also be assessed by measuring the oxygen saturation of a digit using a pulse oximeter. While these give an accurate assessment of skin circulation it is possible to have muscle ischaemia in the presence of a normal skin circulation. Ischaemic muscle is painful if stretched and so a full passive range of movement of a joint distal to a suspected injury excludes it if sensation is intact and the patient is fully conscious. A normal circulation distal to a supracondylar fracture of the humerus can be described as:

'Radial pulse normal
Normal colour, temperature, capillary return < 1 sec
sO$_2$ in finger 97%
Full passive movements of wrist/fingers'

Arterial injuries should be suspected deep to any wound which overlies an artery. A history of pulsatile blood loss should raise suspicions of such an injury but neither its absence nor a normal circulation distal to the wound as determined by an examination as detailed above, will exclude an arterial wound and so any wound in which an arterial injury is a significant possibility should be formally explored or investigated by angiography.

In a compartment syndrome the blood supply to the muscles within a compartment of a limb is reduced because of raised intracompartment pressure caused by bleeding, oedema etc. Although the circulation to the skin should be looked at as should the sensation to the skin (as there may be nerve ischaemia) this may be normal. The signs to look for specifically and to record are tenseness of the compartment to palpation and the presence of pain on stretching the muscles of the compartment. For example in the footballer who has been kicked on the calf, who has severe pain in the absence of a bony injury, the notes might read:

'Bruising calf, feels tense, full painless ankle movement
Sensation, capillary return, temperature of toes all normal
Diagnosis: bruised calf—no evidence compartment syndrome'

or

'Bruising calf, feels tense, foot held in plantar flexion
Pain + + on passive dorsiflexion
Sensation, capillary return, temperature of toes all normal
Diagnosis: ? compartment syndrome—refer orthopaedic surgeons.'

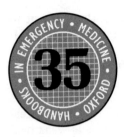

CHAPTER 35

Nerve injury

Key points in nerve injury
- Any wound overlying a nerve must be assumed to have injured it until proved otherwise.
- *Altered* sensation within a nerve distribution indicates that the nerve is divided unless it can be shown to be uninjured at surgery.

Nerve injuries occur within the spinal cord, at nerve roots, in the plexuses, and in peripheral nerves; and the examination is different for suspected injuries at each level. Thus to exclude a nerve root lesion in a patient with neck pain one needs to examine at least one muscle group supplied by each root from C5 to T1 and the sensation within each dermatome (see Chapter 18). The neurological examination for a peripheral nerve injury should look at the motor power and sensation in the areas supplied by any nerve which could be injured. Between the roots and the nerves is the brachial plexus where an injury will produce a different pattern of signs. *A basic knowledge of the anatomy of the nervous system is essential for clinical examination and record keeping in A&E departments.*

Peripheral nerve injury: Examination

Peripheral nerves can be divided in a wound and injured by a fracture, dislocation or external pressure (e.g. the radial nerve 'Saturday night palsy'. Patients may also present to A&E with symptoms due to nerve entrapment (e.g. carpal tunnel syndrome).

The muscles supplied by the nerves most commonly injured are shown in Table 35.1 and clearly the muscles tested to exclude an injury will depend on the level of injury. As an initial screening test for motor weakness it is only necessary to test a single muscle but if power in this is weak or if there is other evidence for a a nerve injury then one should test other muscles supplied by the same nerve. For a median nerve injury at the level of the elbow, examine motor power in flexor pollicis longus or flexor digitorum profundus to the index finger. A wrist laceration is distal to the origin of these muscles and so to exclude an injury at this level, power should be tested in abductor pollicis brevis or opponens pollicis. Sensation is tested on the palmar aspect of the thumb, index, and middle fingers. When testing sensation in any nerve distribution one should always ask the question 'Does that feel normal?' or 'Does it feel the same in all the fingers?' as the answer to the question 'Can you feel that?' will almost always be 'Yes' even if the nerve is completely divided. Radial nerve injuries at the elbow will cause weakness of wrist and finger extension but division at the wrist will cause no weakness. Radial nerve sensory loss is tested over a small area on the dorsum of the hand at the base of the thumb. For an ulna nerve injury, one should examine motor power in the interossei and abductor digiti minimi and sensation in the little finger and ulna side of the ring finger.

Examples of notes on a possible nerve injury

For a severe laceration at the elbow the notes could read:

'Median n √ Ulna n √ Radial n √'

but on the principle that one should record what one has actually done, it is better to write:

Table 35.1 • Main muscles supplied by the peripheral nerves

Radial nerve Triceps
Brachioradialis
All the wrist, thumb and finger extensors
Abductor pollicis longus

Median nerve
Flexor carpi radialis
Flexor pollicis longus
Flexor digitorum superficialis
Flexor digitorum profundus to the index and middle fingers
1st and 2nd lumbricals
Thenar muscles abductor pollicis brevis
                flexor pollicis brevis
                opponens pollicis

Ulna nerve
Flexor carpi ulnaris
Flexor digitorum profundus to the little and ring fingers
All the intrinsic muscles of the hand excluding the thenar muscles
described under the median nerve i.e.
  all the interossei
  3rd and 4th lumbricals
  all muscles of the hypothenar eminence
  flexor pollicis brevis and adductor pollicis

Femoral nerve
Quadriceps
Iliopsoas

Obturator nerve
Hip adductors

Sciatic nerve
Gluteals
Hamstrings
Part of adductor magnus

Divisions of sciatic nerve
Lateral popliteal nerve (and branches)
  tibialis anterior
  peroneals
  toe extensors

Medial popliteal nerve (and branches)
  gastrocnemius and soleus
  tibialis posterior
  long toe flexors
  most of the intrinsic muscles of the foot

'Median n   FDS to index √
Ulna n   Ab Dig Min √
Radial n   Ext Dig √
Sensation   intact in all areas
—no evidence nerve injury'

Whereas for a wrist laceration one could write eg:

'Median n Abd Poll Br √
Ulna n   Abd Dig Min—3/5
                 Interossei—3/5
Sensation present in all fingers but altered in little finger and ulna side ring finger both sides.—ulna nerve injury'

Unfortunately, in a child or on examination of nerve function distal to a displaced and very painful fracture it may not be possible to do an ideal nerve examination. For further examples of notes see Chapter 24.

In the leg the common nerve to be injured is the sciatic nerve (in posterior hip dislocation) and its branches (in injuries around the knee). Examples of appropriate notes in posterior hip dislocation would be:

'Normal power in ankle, normal sensation lower leg'

or, for a laceration at the back of the knee:

'Lat. Pop. n. ankle dorsiflexion √
                  sensation dorsum √
Med. Pop. n. ankle plantar flexion √
                  sensation sole √'

Bracial plexus injuries

A diagram of the brachial plexus is shown in Fig. 35.1. From this it will be seen that to define fully the location and extent of a brachial plexus injury it is necessary to to do a full examination of the nerve roots and of the peripheral nerves. In addition one needs to examine other nerves (e.g. the suprascapular nerve supplying supra- and infraspinatus) which would not be part of a routine neurological examination. However these patients often have other significant

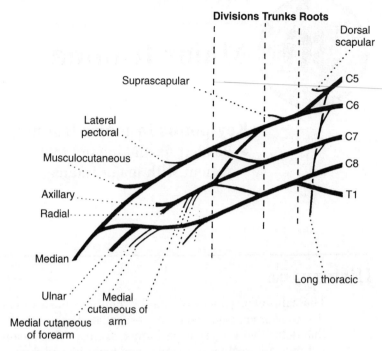

Fig. 35.1 • Simpified diagram of the brachial plexus.

injuries and a definitive examination can be done as an inpatient. In A&E, apart from the routine examination of each root and peripheral nerve as previously described it is necessary to examine the eye for a Horner's syndrome which would indicate a T1 root lesion and to examine the circulation to the upper limb (see Chapter 34) to exclude a subclavian artery injury which is commonly associated with a plexus palsy.

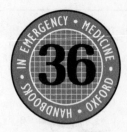

CHAPTER 36

Major trauma

Key points in major trauma
- Be alert for the missed injury in the patient with major trauma.

History

The safe management of life-threatening injuries demands that they are recognized early, resuscitated aggressively, and that definitive surgery is performed rapidly. This means that patients are treated by a senior and experienced doctor. Unfortunately, life-threatening injuries may not always be immediately obvious. Various studies have investigated the mechanisms which are likely to predict serious injury, and in the United States protocols have been drawn up to provide criteria for transporting patients to a trauma centre rather than to the nearest hospital. Details vary but a typical protocol which includes the mechanisms suggesting major injury is shown in Table 36.1. In the UK these patients will normally be taken to the nearest A&E department. Many will not have a life threatening injury, despite the major forces involved, but in view of the association between these factors and significant injury these criteria should be used for calling a trauma team or for the primary survey to be done by an experienced doctor. These criteria will need to be specifically asked about and their presence or absence noted.

On receiving a seriously injured patient into an A&E department the priority is the primary survey but there should

Table 36.1 • **Indications for calling the trauma team**

Mechanisms of injury
  1 Motor vehicle accident > 40 mph
  2 Pedestrian hit by vehicle > 20 mph
  3 Ejection from vehicle
  4 Vehicle roll over
  5 Another occupant of vehicle killed in accident
  6 Fall from height > 20 ft

Anatomical factors
  7 Penetrating injury to head, neck, chest, abdomen, pelvis, or groin
  8 Two or more proximal long bone fractures

Physiological factors
  9 Blood pressure < 100 mmHg
 10 Respiratory rate > 29 or < 10 per minute
 11 Glasgow Coma Score < 11

still be time to ask the patient (if conscious): 'what happened?' and to ask the ambulance personnel the three brief but essential questions:

'What happened?
What treatment has been given?
What change has there been in the patient's condition?'

However, much more history will be required. Most serious trauma is the result of road traffic accidents or falls and details of the history required for these are given in Chapter 37. The history which should be recorded for individual injuries is described in specific chapters. This full description of the accident should be obtained during the secondary survey but too often the ambulance crew has, by then, been called away to another incident. The ambulance report form should contain the essential patient details (e.g. times, vital signs on scene, treatment given etc.), and must be read and should become part of the A&E record. It is not, however, a substitute for talking to witnesses and someone should be delegated to collect the information before the ambulance crew leave. If important points in the history need to be clarified after witnesses have left, an attempt should be made to speak to them by telephone and such calls should be documented.

Details of past medical history, medication etc. should always be enquired about and details of when the patient last ate or drank (and what) may assist the anaesthetist. A helpful mnemonic is that one should take an AMPLE history:[1]

Allergies
Medication
Past medical history
Last ate and drank
Events (i.e. the mechanism of injury etc.)

The weight of a child should be enquired about as this may affect fluid replacement regimes and drug doses.

Examination

Trauma is the commonest cause of death in young people. Its management may be difficult and numerous studies have shown that preventable deaths occur. It is important therefore to audit the care given by reviewing the notes for preventable causes of morbidity and mortality. It is equally important that outcomes are audited. The standard method uses the TRISS methodology[2] which predicts outcome based on the anatomical severity of the injury (Injury Severity Score), physiological variables on arrival (the Revised Trauma Score) and the age of the patient. The Revised Trauma Score is calculated from the Glasgow Coma Score, systolic blood pressure and respiratory rate and so these must be noted on arrival. As these three physiological measures may also be used as criteria for calling more senior help (see Table 36.1), it is essential they are noted for every patient. It is important that patients receive definitive treatment for their injuries within the 'golden hour' after injury, time of arrival into and departure from the department should be noted as should other times, such as the time to establish a clear airway and the times of arrival of key senior staff and specialists.

It is important that major trauma is managed systematically and the standard way of doing this is by following the principles laid down by the Advanced Trauma Life Support (ATLS) course of the American College of Surgeons.[1] It is not the only system for managing major trauma, and some hospitals may modify parts of it, but the basic principles are almost universally accepted. The system divides the management of major trauma into four phases:

1. Primary survey
2. Resuscitation phase
3. Secondary survey
4. Definitive care phase

The first three phases may be done in the A&E department.

The primary survey consists of the identification of life threatening problems and their correction. This is done in strict order:

Airway maintainance with cervical spine control
Breathing and ventilation
Circulation with haemorrhage control
Disability: neurological status
Exposure: completely undress the patient to allow for a full secondary survey

It is useful if the notes of the findings on examination and the management of a patient with major injuries are kept in the same **ABCDE** pattern.

Under the airway, note should be made of any finding on examination which would suggest the possibility of airway problems (e.g. coma, facial injuries, foreign material, including blood, in the pharynx), evidence of actual airway obstruction (e.g. noisy respiration, poor airflow), and the methods used to clear the airway (e.g. airways, suction, cricothyroidotomy). Note should also be made of the measures taken to protect the cervical spine e.g.

'**A**—Airway clear, cervical collar *in situ*, sandbags/tape to stabilize head'

or

'**A**—Obvious # mandible, comatose, blood in pharynx
Chin lift, jaw thrust, oropharygeal airway, suction
Clear airway established
Firm collar applied, sandbags/tape'

or

'**A** — Comatose head injury, jaw tightly closed, obvious airway obstruction with noisy breathing and excessive chest movement
Would not tolerate oropharyngeal airway
Nasopharygeal airway — helped but airway still not clear, so: cricothyroidotomy performed (transverse incision size 6 tracheostomy tube)
Firm collar, manual in-line immobilization of neck'

Under-breathing, evidence of chest injury (e.g. wounds, bruises, flail chest, evidence of a pneumothorax) and the adequacy of ventilation (e.g. respiratory rate, the presence of cyanosis, the oxygen saturation as measured on a pulse oximeter, blood gases) should be noted together with details of procedures done to correct problems found e.g.

'**B** — seat belt bruise chest, no respiratory distress
RR 18, chest clear, slightly tender sternum,
sO_2 (on air) 97%, O_2 given by mask'

or

'**B** — Obvious respiratory distress, cyanosed, RR 40, sO_2 75%
Obvious central flail, surgical emphysema on left
Breath sounds L = R
O_2 by mask
Anaesthetist called, urgent CXR'

or

'**B** — Obviously short of breath, RR 32, tender left chest
Trachea → R, breath sound on left
Clinically tension pneumothorax
Needle decompression left 2nd ICS, MCL some air came out and some improvement
Chest drain 32Fr left 5th ICS, AAL much air came out and 200 ml blood
Afterwards RR 26, sO_2 99% (on oxygen)'

Undercirculation should be recorded evidence of shock (pulse, BP, skin colour, capillary return) and its causes (e.g. exsanguinating haemorrhage or cardiac tamponade). As with the airway and breathing, note should also be made of any treatment given at this stage (e.g. fluid replacement, pericardial aspiration, splinting of limbs to control haemorrhage). Because setting up an intravenous infusion allows blood to be taken and sent for laboratory analyses this should be noted at this stage. Examples of notes are:

'C—Obvious bleeding from laceration over left brachial artery
Direct pressure applied
P 120 (regular but weak), BP 55/? pale, sweaty, slow capillary return (5 secs)
IVI right antecubital fossa
Cut down left long saphenous vein
Bloods taken for FBC
   U&E
   XM 6 units'

or (e.g. in a patient with crush injuries to the lower limbs)

'C—P 100 (regular), BP 100/60
IVI × 2 (both antecubital fossae)
Blood for FBC
   U&E
   XM 6 units
Donway splints both legs
ECG monitor (sinus tachy)'

The assessment of disability is a brief examination of the central nervous system with an assessment of the level of consciousness and the pupils. The ATLS system teaches that the Glasgow Coma Score (GCS) should be measured in the secondary survey and that at this early stage, the level of consciousness should be rapidly assessed using the 'AVPU' method, i.e.

Alert
Responds to Vocal stimuli
Responds to Painful stimuli
Unresponsive

However, it takes little longer to measure the GCS, and as discussed above, this should be done on arrival both as a means of triage and as a baseline for audit purposes. The assessment of conscious level may also reveal evidence of spinal cord injury (e.g. movement of the arms but not the legs to painful stimuli) or localizing signs (e.g. one side moves more than the other). These can be noted at this point. A full description of the level of consciousness as described in Chapter 16 can be done during the secondary survey. Examples of the notes which could be made at this stage include:

'**D**—GCS 15, PERL'

or

'**D**—GCS V = 2, E = 2, M = 4 (left side moves less than right)
    Left pupil normal, reacts to light
    Right pupil dilated, no reaction'

The resuscitation phase of management will normally be documented by the nursing notes with charts of volumes and types of fluid replacement and vital signs. However vital signs should be noted at intervals in the medical notes, especially where patient management decisions have been based on them e.g.

'1405 hr P 100, BP 105/60, Hartman's solution 500 ml × 2 given 1420 hr P 110, BP 90/60, 2 units blood stat, surgeons called'

The vital signs when the patient leaves the department should be noted and it is also useful to summarize the total fluid repacement given until that time e.g.

'Total fluid given: prehospital   500 ml saline
                      A&E   1500 ml saline
                                1000 ml haemaccel
                                   2 U O neg blood'

The ATLS system also teaches that urinary catheters and nasogastric or orogastric tubes should be inserted during the resuscitation phase if there is no contraindication. The size of catheter, volume, and colour of urine should all be noted.

If a patient has a very painful injury, it is easy to overlook or play down the importance of another less painful but possibly more serious injury elsewhere. If there are two injuries in the same limb it is common to miss the more proximal injury as, for example, one cannot fully move and examine the hip in the presence of a fractured tibia. Injuries are even more likely to be missed if the patient has a diminished level of consciousness because of a head injury or intoxication or if they have loss of pain sensation due to e.g. a spinal cord injury. This is obviously of great importance if a life-threatening injury is not to be missed (e.g. an abdominal injury missed in a comatose patient who cannot complain of tenderness) but it is also important that minor injuries are not overlooked. A flexor tendon injury to a finger will initially have a lower priority for treatment in a patient who also has a flail chest and a ruptured spleen but its prognosis is best when treated within the first 24 hours and if not properly treated it may cause a major handicap. If there is a conscious decision to give priority to more serious problems, secondary tendon repair may be the optimal management but delayed treatment because the injury was initially overlooked is unacceptable. Road accidents and falls are likely to cause more than one injury and so every patient who has been involved in such an accident or who has been exposed to major forces must have a head to toe examination (including the back). This is called the *secondary survey*. Thus, a patient involved in a road accident who has has a minor head injury may have a secondary survey noted as:

$$
\left.
\begin{array}{l}
\text{neck} \\
\text{spine} \\
\text{chest} \\
\text{abdomen} \\
\text{pelvis} \\
\text{arms} \\
\text{legs}
\end{array}
\right\} \quad \text{all NAD}
$$

However, this does not indicate what exact examination has been done and it would be better to record more detail such as:

neck: not tender, full painless ROM
spine: not tender
chest: not tender, no pain on springing chest, breath sounds L = R = NAD

abdomen: no tenderness, guarding, rebound. BS normal
pelvis: no pain on springing
legs: no tenderness, full ROM all joints, normal gait
arms: no tenderness, full ROM

If an abnormality is found in a system, note keeping should be as described in the relevent chapter although this is not always possible because of the patient's clinical state.

When a patient leaves the A&E department it is important that their injuries are listed and this includes not just the diagnosed injuries but those which are suspected. Injuries must be described fully to allow an accurate calculation of the Injury Severity Score. A note must also be made of what aspects of the examination it was not possible to do and therefore what injuries were not excluded. For example in a patient being transferred immediately to theatre the diagnosis might read:

'*Diagnosis*:
1 Head injury, right extradural haematoma
2 Fractures left 4th and 5th ribs laterally
3 Clinical closed fracture right tibia—splinted—not yet X-rayed
4 NB back not yet examined'

or (in another patient)

'1 Head injury GCS 11 SXR & CT normal
2 C7/T1 not seen on XR so keep in firm collar, reX-ray mane
3 Transverse laceration anterior aspect right wrist 5 cm long—tendons, nerves not examined because of diminished level of consciousness'

If a patient has multiple fractures, these can be well demonstrated on a chart such as shown in Fig. 36.1.

Once the patient has been resuscitated, the most senior doctor involved must speak to the patient's relatives. A brief description of what has been said, particularly as regards any prognosis given, is important for the next person who needs to speak to them. This note can be fairly brief e.g.

'Spoke to wife and son, told them that he has a severe head injury and that he is unlikely to survive'

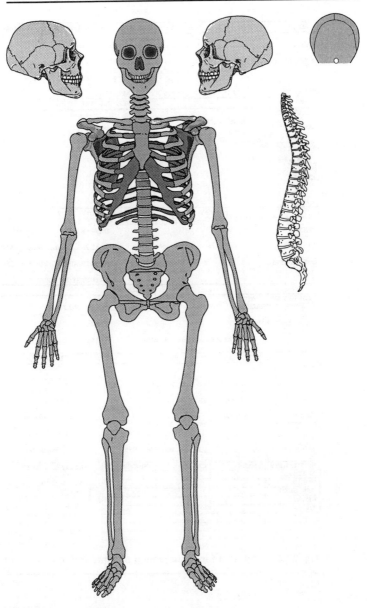

Fig. 36.1 • Chart for documenting fractures.

```
ACCIDENT & EMERGENCY , DERRIFORD HOSPITAL , PLYMOUTH.        TRAUMA CHART

NAME..........................        COMPLETED BY.....................

ADDRESS.......................        DATE............................

..............................        TIME OF ARRIVAL........

AGE\DOB......... A&E No..........     A&E DRS..........................
HISTORY                               PREHOSPITAL CARE
ALLERGIES

MEDICATION

PAST ILLNESS

LAST ATE OR DRANK

EVENTS


                  AIRWAY WITH CERVICAL SPINE PROTECTION
                     RIGID COLLAR/SANDBAGS/HEAD TAPES
PATENT                                OXYGEN          L/MINUTE

AT RISK                               ORAL/NASOPHARYNGEAL AIRWAY

OBSTRUCTED                            ENDOTRACHEAL TUBE SIZE....

                                      CRICOTHYROIDOTOMY
                           BREATHING
RESPIRATORY RATE
            TRACHEA                   CHEST DRAINS

            AIR ENTRY                 SIZE........

     O2 SATURATION...%on...l/minO2    SIZE........

        CIRCULATION                            DISABILITY
BLOOD PRESSURE                        G.C.S.
            IVI 1 SITE ......GAUGE....    E
            IVI 2 SITE ......GAUGE....
            IVI 3 SITE ......GAUGE....    M

PULSE       BLOOD    O NEG                V
                     GROUP & SAVE
                     X MATCH.....UNITS    TOTAL

                     BLOOD WARMER  Y/N       PUPILS
```

SPECIALITY	GRADE	CALLED	ARRIVED
ANAESTH.			
ORTHO.			
GEN.SURG.			
NEURO.			
THORACIC			
PLASTIC			

```
INITIAL X-RAYS

LAT.C-SPINE
(?C7/T1)

CHEST
(ERECT IF POS)

PELVIS
```

Fig. 36.2 • Proforma for documenting patients with major trauma.

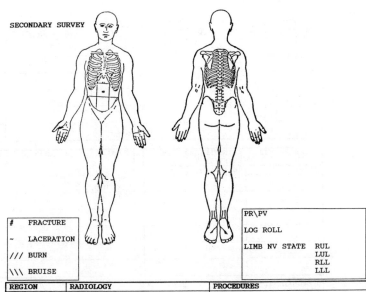

SECONDARY SURVEY

#	FRACTURE		
~	LACERATION		
///	BURN		
\\\	BRUISE		

PR\PV

LOG ROLL

LIMB NV STATE   RUL
                 LUL
                 RLL
                 LLL

REGION	RADIOLOGY	PROCEDURES
HEAD & NECK	CT HEAD SKULL XRAY	
THORAX	ERECT CXR	ECG(12 lead) CVP PERICARDIOCENTESIS
ABDOMEN	CT ABDOMEN ULTRASOUND IVP	NASOGASTRIC TUBE OROGASTRIC TUBE URINARY CATHETER SIZE... PERITONEAL LAVAGE
SPINE	C.SPINE SERIES T.SPINE SERIES L.SPINE SERIES	
EXTREMITIES		SPLINTAGE

IVI 1	SITE			IVI 2	SITE		
TIME	FLUID	VOLUME	TOTAL	TIME	FLUID	VOLUME	TOTAL
TOTAL				TOTAL			

URINE OUTPUT	CATHETERISED Y/N URINE TEST		DRUGS	SIGNATURE	GIVEN BY
TIME	TOTAL DRAINED				
			TETANUS TOXOID 0.5 ML		
			HATI 250U		

DISPOSAL	TO	AT	HRS	GCS	Bp	/	P	RR

RESULTS	TIME	TIME
pO2		
pCO2		
pH		
Na		
K		
Urea		
Bicarb.		
Hb		
WCC		
Plats.		
Gluc.		
Amylase		

SUMMARY OF INJURIES

DEFINITE

SUSPECTED

NOT EXCLUDED

GSJ 11/93 A&E DEPT

GLASGOW COMA SCORE	TIME	HRS MINS																		
EYE OPENING.	SPONTANEOUS	4																		
	TO SPEECH	3																		
	TO PAIN	2																		
	NONE	1																		
BEST MOTOR RESPONSE	OBEYS COMMANDS	6																		
	LOCALISES	5																		
	WITHDRAWS	4																		
	FLEXION TO PAIN	3																		
	EXTENSION TO PAIN	2																		
	NONE	1																		
BEST VERBAL RESPONSE	ORIENTATED	5																		
	CONFUSED	4																		
	INAPPROPRIATE	3																		
	INCOMPREHENSIBLE	2																		
	NONE	1																		
TOTAL																				

PUPILS	SIZE	RIGHT																		
		LEFT																		
	REACTION	RIGHT																		
		LEFT																		
LIMB POWER	UPPER	RIGHT																		
		LEFT																		
	LOWER	RIGHT																		
		LEFT																		

Pupil scale (m.m.)
• 1
● 2
● 3
● 4
● 5
● 6
● 7
● 8

BLOOD PRESSURE	220																		
	210																		
	190																		
	180																		
	170																		
	160																		
	150																		
	140																		
	130																		
	120																		
PULSE	110																		
	100																		
	90																		
	80																		
	70																		
	60																		
	50																		
	40																		
	30																		
RESPIRATION RATE	20																		
	10																		
	0																		

TEMPERATURE																			
PULSE OXIMETRY																			

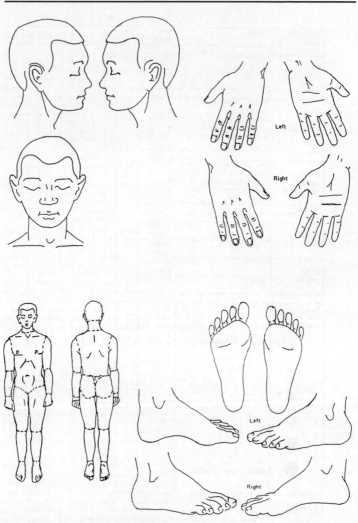

Fig. 36.3 · Chart for documenting wounds.

or

'Spoke with parents, told them that Ian has severe injuries but he has good prognostic signs and so will probably be all right but cannot guarantee that he will survive'

The management of patients with major injuries may be difficult, with many people involved and a great sense of urgency. The quality of note keeping may suffer. For this reason it is useful to have a proforma or chart to collect essential information on such patients. An example of such is shown in Fig. 36.2. The use of a proforma has also been shown to improve not only the note keeping (which should itself improve clinical care) but also the standard of clinical care,[3] as it prevents doctors forgetting aspects of the examination, investigation, and management. The information gathered on this type of proforma must, however, only be regarded as a minimum as additional data will need to be collected and notes made. For example, the diagram of the body is too small to accurately describe the position of wounds on the hands and face. If there are injuries to these areas, notes will need to be made as described in the relevant chapters. A chart for more accurately describing wounds is shown in Fig. 36.3.

References

1. American College of Surgeons (1989). *Advanced trauma life support course*. American College of Surgeons, Chicago, Illinois, USA.
2. Boyd, C. R., Tolson, M. A., and Copes, W. S. (1987). Evaluating trauma care: the TRISS method. *Journal of Trauma*, **27**, 370–78.
3. Murat, J. E., Huten, N., and Mesny, J. (1986). The use of standardised assessment procedures in the evaluation of patients with multiple injuries. *Archives of Emergency Medicine*, **2**, 11–15.

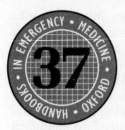

CHAPTER 37

Road traffic
accidents and falls

History

'RTA' as the only history appearing on the A&E record is inadequate. Injuries are caused by forces acting on the human body and it is important to estimate the size and direction of those forces and to know what restraining methods were used (e.g. seat belts, air bags). Estimates of speed may be inaccurate but an assessment of the damage to the vehicle (e.g. the amount of intrusion of the doors or roof and the integrity of the frame) will give a good indication of the forces involved and provide valuable clues to the types of injury to be expected. In general terms, the greater the force acting on the body, the greater is the likelihood of serious injury. Specific details of the accident may raise the suspicion of specific injuries. For example, the crumpled steering wheel may cause a flail chest; the lap seat belt commonly found in the rear centre seat may cause abdominal injury and the foot tangled beneath the pedals may suffer a midtarsal or tarsometatarsal dislocation. It must not be forgotten that on occasion an accident may be caused by a medical condition (e.g. a myocardial infarction or a fit), and in certain circumstances the physical injuries caused by the initial impact may be complicated by near-drowning, chemical contamination, or burns.

Factors from the history which make the presence of a serious injury likely and which should thus be used as criteria for calling for a trauma team or a senior doctor are given in Table 36.1 (p. 189). Some of these are obvious but others (e.g. the death of a patient in an accident being an indicator that others in the same accident have a high chance of serious injury) will need to be specifically considered.

All A&E staff find it difficult to remember all the details which need to be asked about a road traffic accident, especially in a patient with major injuries when the primary survey takes priority and the detailed history is left to a very junior doctor or nurse. To assist in obtaining this information the mnemonic TRAFFIC has been developed (R. Snook, personal communication):

Transfer of forces
Relative direction of impact
Aspect of the vehicle damaged
Focus of force
Frame integrity (car frame)
Intrusion of the car body into the car (and how much)
Contact point

With training, the ambulance personnel can observe and note these details at the scene of the accident without increasing on scene time. These details can be documented on the form shown in Fig. 37.1 either by the ambulance crew or following questioning of them by hospital staff.

Another method of recording the accident is by means of a polaroid photograph taken by the ambulance crew. While this will not document all the information gathered by the chart in Fig. 37.1, it is complementary and in a patient with seemingly minor injuries, a photograph of the wrecked car in which he was travelling will prompt a further search for occult injuries.

In cycle and motor cycle accidents the same type of information should be obtained and the helmet should be inspected to give further clues to the forces acting on the head.

Fall from a height

History

In addition to the usual information to be collected, the following history should be obtained:

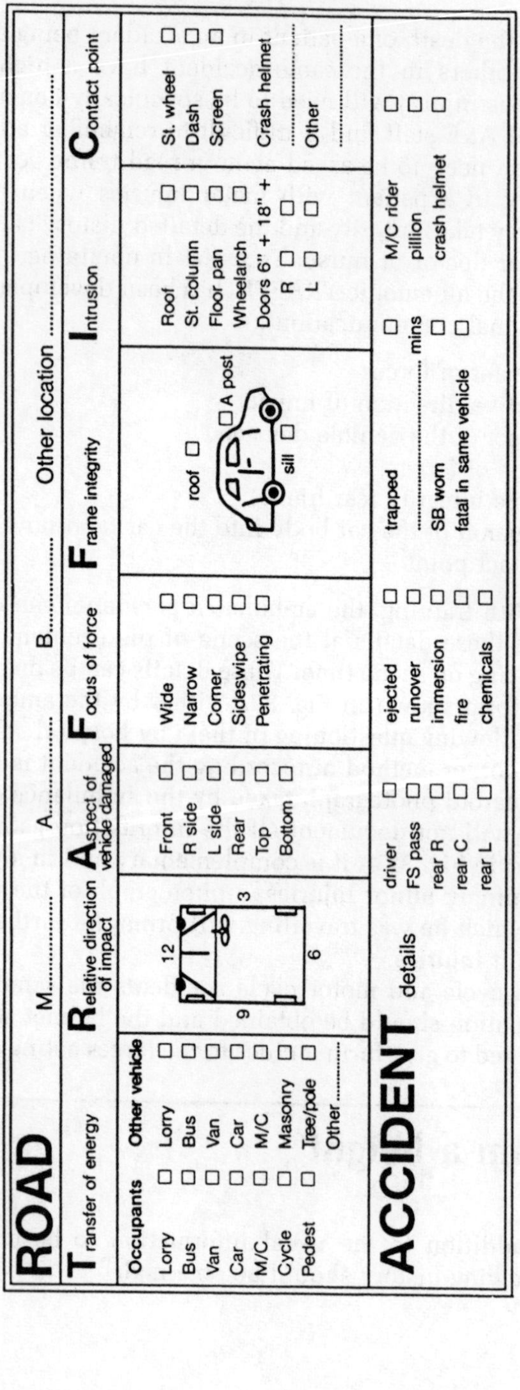

Fig. 37.1 • Chart for obtaining history of patients in road accidents.
(Reproduced by courtesy of Dr R. Snook, Consultant in A&E, Royal United Hospital, Bath.)

- Reason for fall.
- Distance fallen.
- Surface landed on (e.g. grass, concrete).
- How landed (e.g. on head, on heels).
- Did patient strike anything while falling.
- Position found on ground.

Examination

Following a road traffic accident or fall (and in other types of trauma such as assault or an explosion) patients are likely to have more than one injury. Those less painful but possibly more serious may be overlooked their importance played down. For this reason every patient involved in a road accident or fall from a height MUST be fully examined from head to toe before being discharged. At the very least this should include palpation of the skull, the whole spine, the abdomen, the pelvis, and all four limbs; the 'springing' of the chest, the movement of the neck and all four limbs and observing the patient's gait if they are going to be discharged. Note keeping for this secondary survey is described in Chapter 36.

Drinking drivers

Following a road traffic accident the police may seek the doctor's permission for the car driver to be asked to provide a specimen of breath or blood to measure alcohol concentration. This permission should not be refused as long as the patient is in a fit state to give consent and that neither providing the specimen nor being asked to provide it will cause the patient any harm. If permission is sought for a patient to provide a specimen, this should be noted together with the doctors response and possibly reasons e.g.

'*0035 hrs*: asked to give permission for patient to give breath specimen to police—permission given'

or

'. . . permission not given, fractured mandible precludes giving breath and # right humerus and IVI left arm precludes giving blood'

or

'. . . permission refused. Patient disorientated and unable to give consent'

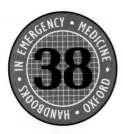

CHAPTER 38

Deliberate self-harm

Key points in deliberate self-harm

- A psychosocial assessment is essential in all cases of deliberate self-harm.

In patients whose injuries are the result of deliberate self-harm the assessment and management of the physical injuries is frequently much easier and faster than sorting out the psychological and social problems underlying the self-harm. However, it is important and a requirement of the Department of Health that a psycho-social history and assessment is carried out. As with physical problems, good record keeping is essential. If a patient has major injuries (e.g. as a result of jumping from a height) the management of the physical injuries will clearly take priority and the assessment can be done later during the inpatient stay. If the injuries are less severe (e.g. lacerations of the arm and wrist) a preliminary assessment must be done in A&E even if the patient is going to be admitted and assessed in detail later. The reason for this is that a severe psychiatric illness may be a greater threat to life and health than their wound and may need to take priority. A practical reason for doing an early assessment is that if the patient wishes to leave without treatment, the doctor must have the evidence to decide whether the patient is well enough to sign a form stating that he discharges himself against medical advice or whether he requires compulsory admission. This is allowed under the Mental Health Act if the patient is suffering from a mental disorder which warrants admission to hospital and he ought to be detained in the interests of his own health or safety or with a view to the protection of other persons.[1] If it is planned to discharge a patient from A&E, a full assessment must always be made.

The basic history should include:

- Why was the attempt made?
- What method was used?
- Was there suicidal intent?
- How does the patient feel now?
- Is there any evidence of psychiatric disease?
- What support does patient have (e.g. family, friends)?
- Past medical history.

Why?

To ask why the patient harmed himself is a question in two parts. There may be underlying reasons, such as family and employment problems and lack of social support, but it is important to discover what happened to the patient in the previous 48 hours to precipitate the self-harm.

What method?

This is usually self-evident but it is important to ascertain that the patient has not taken an drug overdose in addition to physically harming himself. Ask also about the consumption of alcohol.

Was there suicidal intent?

The severity of the wound (or other injury) does not reflect the seriousness of the psychiatric problem or of the suicidal intent. Rather than asking the direct question 'Did you intend to commit suicide?' to which many patients will routinely answer 'Of course', it is better to ask a more open question such as 'What did you expect to happen?'. It is also important to enquire from the patient (and from others) whether a suicide note was left. Enquiry should also be made as to whether the patient took any precautions against being discovered or whether they immediately sought help. Cutting your wrists in the A&E waiting room may be evidence of psychiatric illness (though is more likely to be highly manipulative behaviour) but it is not an attempt at suicide.

How does the patient feel now?

The patient's present state should be enquired about and noted as part of the assessment as to whether they are suicidal. Examples of questions to ask are:

'Are you sorry you failed to kill yourself?'

and

'Do you still have thoughts of harming/killing yourself?'

Is there any evidence of psychiatric disease?

Past psychiatric illness, admissions, and treatment must obviously be asked about. Psychiatric symptoms may have been apparent at an earlier stage of the history but if not, ask specifically about depression and other symptoms of a depressive illness such as sleep disturbance and feelings of worthlessness.

Past medical history

Past psychiatric problems including previous episodes of overdose or self-harm are obviously important to note. Alcohol and drug abuse should also be asked about. It is also vital to note physical disease as the presence of severe illness is a strong risk factor for future suicide.

The casualty officer is not expected to be a psychiatrist but as when dealing with any patient, it is important to establish a diagnosis. In addition, using the evidence obtained during the psycho-social history and knowledge of other risk factors such as the patient's age, sex etc. an assessment should be made of the risk of suicide or of further attempts at self harm. Finally a decision as to how the patient can be best helped should be made and recorded.

Examples of notes on self-harm

History from son:
(patient withdrawn and not communicating)
Widowed 2 years ago
Appeared well this a.m. Son came home from work early and found a suicide note Went to bathroom, had to batter the door down, and found father in bath with cut wrists. Depressed since he lost his job 4/12 ago. Has mentioned suicide but light-heartedly and no-one took it seriously.
Not seen GP.
PMH: Nil significant, no psychiatric illness, no medication.
Diagnosis: severe depression, significant suicide risk.
Plan: admit. If he tries to self discharge he will need urgent psychiatric assessment for ? sectioning.

or

History from patient:
Lives at home with parents. Works in factory.
Girlfriend walked out on him and he went and had a few drinks and then went and sat on her doorstep and cut his wrists with a razor blade. Says it was impulsive.
Says he wanted to die but now regrets action and says he feels stupid.
No wish to kill himself now.
Has good friends, plays football 2 × per week.
PMH:
Nil significant, no psychiatric illness or overdoses
No depression, sleeps well.
Alcohol: consumes 7–8 units once or twice a week, never done anything stupid under influence of alcohol before.
Assessment: impulsive behaviour under the influence of alcohol, no evidence of psychiatric illness or suicide risk.
Plan: Will go and see GP tomorrow.
Letter to GP given to patient and copy posted.

Reference

1. Bluglass, R. (1983). *A guide to the Mental Health Act 1983.* Churchill Livingstone, Edinburgh.

PART 5

The nurse's contribution towards note taking

A. M. JENKINS

39 Nurse's notes

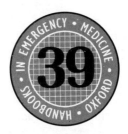

CHAPTER 39

Nurse's notes

What is asked today—might be forgotten tomorrow

The United Kingdom Central Council (1993),[1] gives clear instructions on the required standards of nursing records and record keeping. Their 'Summary of the principles underpinning the records and record keeping' is shown on p. 218.

Triage and initial assessment

The notes of the initial assessment should contain a history of the patients' perceived problem, and observations of the patients' condition or injury. It should also contain a brief but concise and accurate account of why the patient has attended the A&E department.

The notes should be recorded in black ink or biro to facilitate photocopying at a later date. The writing should be clear, without spelling mistakes, and signed by the nurse undertaking the assessment. If your signature is not clear it is essential to print your name beneath.

It is necessary to have full details of the patients' injury in order to triage the patient, but remember that the patient will be asked similar questions by the doctor and too much repetition should be avoided. However, many junior doctors in A&E may be less experienced than the triage nurse and if significant abnormalities are found they should be highlighted. For example:

1601 hrs:
Laceration to Left Index finger, on a metal shelf at work
half an hour ago. Would approx 1.5 cm., on medial aspect.
Patient can't flex DIP joint.
? Tendon injury.
Temporary dry dressing applied.
Tetanus UTD, < 3 years.   (signed) *I. S. Clear*
1604 hrs:

Abbreviations, if used, should be locally recognized.

Documenting the time at all stages is important, not only
for audit but for chronological record of the care received
and by whom. By reviewing the A&E record we should be
able to plot the course of the patients visit to the department
in detail. See Fig. 39.1.

Documentation of care should be done as soon as that care
has been given, but there are occasions when an emergency
requires immediate intervention and documentation is deferred. If at all possible delegate this task to a colleague from
the start. This enables an accurate account to be made. A
delay in recording details, however short, allows omissions
and inconsistencies.

Similarly, if the nurse is suspicious that what are presented as accidents or injuries were caused by some other
mechanism (e.g. assault or self-harm), this should be noted
to warn others who will see the patient. To wait until the
doctor has formulated a treatment plan and explained it to
the patient and parents before raising a suspicion of an NAI,
is to wait too long.

By carefully listening to the ambulance personnel or relatives and recording all observations and details, mistakes
can be prevented. For example, the GP may have given prehospital analgesia and in his haste, written it out on the back
of an envelope which was discarded.

On occasion a patient may not wait to see the doctor—but
could return to A&E or complain that he or she was not
treated on his initial visit. Accurate notes made by the triage
nurse will demonstrate that the patient was not abandoned
and that the nurse did not deny the patient access to medical
advice. If the patient becomes verbally abusive when in-

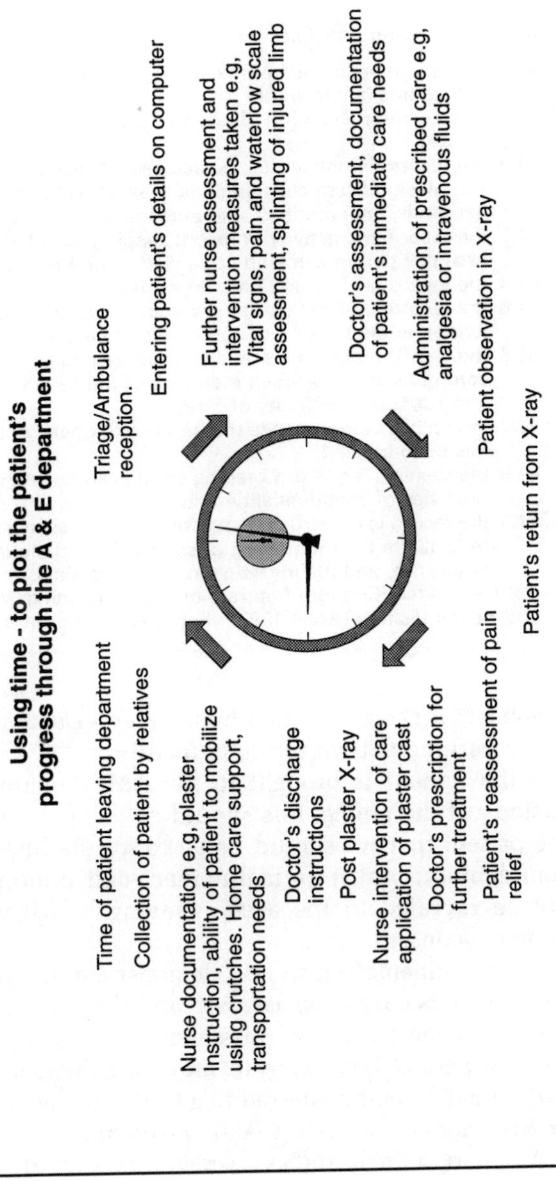

Using time - to plot the patient's progress through the A & E department

Triage/Ambulance reception.

Entering patient's details on computer

Further nurse assessment and intervention measures taken e.g, Vital signs, pain and waterlow scale assessment, splinting of injured limb

Doctor's assessment, documentation of patient's immediate care needs

Administration of prescribed care e.g, analgesia or intravenous fluids

Patient observation in X-ray

Patient's return from X-ray

Patient's reassessment of pain relief

Doctor's prescription for further treatment

Nurse intervention of care application of plaster cast

Post plaster X-ray

Doctor's discharge instructions

Nurse documentation e.g, plaster Instruction, ability of patient to mobilize using crutches. Home care support, transportation needs

Collection of patient by relatives

Time of patient leaving department

Fig. 39.1 • Time-plotting the patient's progress through A&E.

Summary of the principles underpinning records and record keeping

41 The following principles must apply:

41.1 the record is directed primary to serving the interests of the patient or client to whom it relates and enabling the provision of care, the prevention of disease, and the promotion of health;

41.2 the record demonstrates the accurate chronology of events and all significant consultations, assessments, observations, decisions, interventions, and outcomes;

41.3 the record and activity of record keeping is an integral and essential part of care and not a distraction from its provision;

41.4 the record is clear and unambiguous;

41.5 the record contains entries recording facts and observations written at the time of, or soon after, the events described;

41.6 the record provides a safe and effective means of communication between members of the health care team and supports continuity of care;

41.7 the record demonstrates that the practitioners' duty of care has been fulfilled;

41.8 the systems for record keeping exclude authorized access and breaches of confidentiality; and

41.9 the record is constructed and completed in such a manner as to facilitate the monitoring of standards, audit, quality assurance, and the investigation of complaints.

Source: United Kingdom Central Council for Nursing, Midwifery and Health Visiting (April, 1993). (Published by permission.)

---

formed that there is a two hour delay—Document it! You will recall the patient far more readily.

If the patient is brought to the A&E department in the custody of the police, this should be recorded but it is still the patient that we should listen to for the history. Patient confidentiality must be maintained, and information must not be revealed to the accompanying police without the patient's consent.

The documentation should demonstrate that the patient's requirements have been assessed and should state the action needed to meet those requirements. For example, lifting— has the patient been able to move him/herself or has the patient had to be transferred to a trolley using an Easy Glide or stretcher canvas, poles, and spreaders.

As a part of the initial assessment one should, in appropriate cases, make use of the Waterlow Measurement Scale.[2] Patients of all ages are susceptible to pressure ulcers if their mobility is restricted for prolonged periods (e.g. The elderly, the unconscious, or patients with a spinal injury).

By recording such an assessment, the patients potential vulnerability is highlighted and nursing staff demonstrate they understand their responsibility to care. The actions taken to prevent further harm (in this example, 'Spenco mattress used', regular turning, and skin condition observations) shoud be noted.

A 10-point analogue pain rating scale can be used to assess the patients level of pain and the nurse can start to implement care by splinting, elevation, and Entonox but full pain relief may not be achieved until the doctor has prescribed analgesia. A further reassessment, using the rating scale, should be done to ensure that the goal of effective pain relief has been achieved. Recording the pain scores is essential for future reassessments.

The nursing record should document relevant information or details that might influence the care and advice offered to the patient. There are many psychological, social, spiritual, and cultural variables that will affect the patient's well-being during his or her stay in the A&E department and each has to be considered.

When a nurse is recording brief details it is appropriate for this information to be written on the A&E record card. However, in patients with more severe medical problems or complex social situations it will often be better to record the information on a specific proforma. This may be ased on a nursing model used in the A&E department or may be designed to correspond to nursing records used on the wards to which patients will be admitted. Such a proforma not only allows easy access to the recorded information but also serves as an *aide-mémoire* to ensure that no relevant details are omitted. An example of a proforma is given in Fig. 39.2.

Observations

We are able to document some observations without using

Plymouth District General Hospital Acute Unit
Accident & Emergency Department, Derriford Hospital
PATIENT ASSESSMENT

Patient's name: N.O.K.
                                         Relationship

Date	Observations: Temp:	Pulse:	BP:	Resp:
Time	Pupils:		Weight:	
	Trauma score:		BM stix:	
	Allergies:		Waterlow score:	

Pain score:

on admission: Post analgesia:

Lifting need on admission:

No. of nurses: Aids:

Method:

History of illness/accident:

Normal state of health & social history:

Current medication:

Fig. 39.2 • Proforma for patient assessment.

Nursing action:

Property & valuables:

Medication given in A & E department:

Condition of patient on discharge:

Name of nurse: Signature:

Discharge plan

Patient discharged to:

Home [ ]   Ward [ ]   Hospital [ ]   NOK. [ ]   Friends [ ]

Other [ ]   Specify:

Follow up:

GP [ ]   District nurse [ ]   Health visitor [ ]

Social worker [ ]   Home help [ ]   Physio [ ]

Other: [ ]   Please specify:

Medication supplied:

Transport required:

Ambulance [ ]   Taxi [ ]   Own [ ]   Other [ ]

Time booked: Arrived:

Name of Nurse: Signature:

any instruments. For example: did the patient hear when called or is the patient communicating by lip-reading? A simple record of 'Hearing impairment—able to lip-read' will save embarrassment when the patient is later called by a colleague.

When a parent informs ou of the child's injury, several observations can be made. Are the child and parent responding well to each other, is the child alert, taking an interest in objects or actively playing with toys or is the child sitting quietly or appearing withdrawn? Make a note on the A&E notes if there is concern or if it is pertinent to the injury. e.g.

'Child fell < 1 hour ago. Small laceration to forehead. Not KO'd, no vomiting. Child is alert and playing with toys. Immunizations UTD'

Is the patient pale, anxious, agitated, smelling of alcohol? Are they unsteady (on their feet) or do they look in pain and distress?

Many patients will need what is often called 'routine observations' recorded. However, these should never be routine. Each patient should be assessed and it is important that initial observations are done early and as the patient is commonly seen first by a nurse, it is usually a nursing responsibility.

It is important to document ALL of the appropriate recordable observations *accurately* and clearly, either on the patient's A&E notes or on a dedicated chart. There should be enough space for the date, time, and a signature to be added. By making a note of our observations we are informing colleagues of our, actions and this can be used to measure changes in the patient's condition and can highlight any potential problems.

Pulse and blood pressure must be recorded on all appropriate patients. The respiratory rate unfortunately is less commonly done in practice but is important and should be done on most 'trolley' patients. Not only is it a valuable way of monitoring patients with respiratory and cardiac problems but it serves as a baseline for patients given respiratory depressant analgesia. In addition, the respiratory rate is an essential measurement for the adult of trauma care (see Chapter 36).

The level of consciousness is also important to record. If the patient has NO history of a head or brain injury and is fully conscious it is enough to say 'alert and orientated', but otherwise the Glasgow Coma Score (GCS), should always be recorded. It is good practice for the nurse who initially recorded the observations to continue with that patient to increase the reliability of the record.

Temperature (including the site and method of measurement) is important in many 'walking wounded' patients with possible sepsis as well as the 'trolley' patients. On occasion additional information gained from this record can influence how we plan our nursing care. For example, for an elderly hypothermic patient we need to consider the effect of body temperature for pressure area care and wound healing.

In patients with limb fractures or injuries that could impede their circulation, the skin colour, temperature, and pulse/s distal to the fracture sites should be documented and compared to the uninjured side, this is recorded as:

Radial pulse: Left = Right
Temperature/colour of hands: Left = Right

If a urine sample is tested the results should be entered on to the patients' notes, together with the volume passed and whether the sample has been saved (in case a further investigation is required). The date and time of the entry should be documented together with a signature of the person making the entry e.g.

23.00 hrs:
Urinalysis, ph 6, NAD, 180 mls.
Sample saved.   *I. S. Clear*

Nurse practitioners

This role has allowed experienced, specialized A&E nurses to undertake their own sphere of practice, to enhance the overall efficiency of the department.

The nurse practitioner should document the history, diagnosis, and treatment plan on the A&E record card in the same manner as his or her medical colleagues. Nurse practitioners are advised to read the relevant chapters in this book. Even if treatment is carried out by a colleague, the nurse practitioner is responsible for that treatment. It is sensible to see the patient following the treatment (e.g. replacing a plaster cast backslab). Not only is the quality and comfort of the plaster cast checked but an opportunity is available to ensure that the patient has heard and understood his plaster instructions.

An example of the record for this patient's attendance would be:

1606 hrs:
Visitor to the area.
Patient attended with a wet plaster backslab, fell in the bath.
Undisplaced fracture left radius 3 weeks ago.
Patient not complaining of any problems related to actual injury.
Treatment 1610 hrs:
Please replace below elbow backslab.
Broad arm sling
Keep fracture clinic appointment on returning to home address.   *I.S. Clear*
1628 hrs:
POP backslab removed, new POP backslab applied to left forearm—neutral position.   *S.E. Nurse*
1640 hrs:
Pop Checked, Instructions understood.
Patient dischard 1642 hrs.   *I.S. Clear*

Specific situations

Violence

If a formalized chart is not available for dealing with a violent patient, careful documentation should be undertaken and should include:

Prehospital information, including:
- Drugs/alcohol.
- Psychiatric history.
- Social history.
- Time of arrival in A.&E.

Description of patients behaviour, including:
- Attempts at communication.
- Type of violence portrayed.
- Threatening behaviour.

Note patient's observable injuries/wounds.

Time police called . . .
Time police arrived . . .

If needed—how and why restrained.
In secure room/observation by:
Physical restraint by police, nurse, security team:
Method of physical restraint.

Time of medical assessment.
Time of notifying social worker.   Name =
Time of notifying psychiatric team.   Name =
Time of notifying hospital manager.   Name =

Time medications given =
What medications given =

Time restraint withdrawn =
Patient's observable behaviour
Ability to communicate with patient
Time of reassessment of patient

Key doctor dealing with event
Key nurse dealing with event

Time patient left department

Evaulation of event/follow-up.

Death

When a patient dies, in the department or is brought in dead, the notes should illustrate what communication has taken place.

Looking after the relatives is often difficult but other hospital services can assist, such as the hospital chaplain or the bereavement officer. Their names should be noted, together with any relevant information they have discovered regarding the patient.

Information regarding prehospital status of the patient is gained from the ambulance personnel or police who accompany the patient. Details of the next of kin (if not present and if known) may need to be passed on to the police so that relatives can be notified.

If the police are contacting relatives, note the policeman's name and number so that when a colleague makes a progress enquiry several hours later, the police controller is able to follow-up the enquiry more swiftly.

If a relative is present in the department document their name, address, telephone number, and relationship to the deceased, so that further enquiries can be dealt with more efficiently.

A rubber stamp is useful to act as a visual reminder of who has been contacted.

Relatives		General practitioner		
Coroner		Social worker		
Police		Health visitor		

Other details to be noted usually relate to specific situations, e.g.

- A social worker may need to be contacted regarding the care of a dependent relative.
- An infant's death may be the result of Sudden Infant Death Syndrome and we need to list the additional investigations done and care given to the parent(s).
  - baptism
  - lock of hair
  - photograph
  - clothing returned (dependent on local police clothing may or may not be able to be returned to the aprent/s.
  - paediatric liaison health visitor contacted

– paediatric social worker contacted.
– paediatric consultant was . . . (name)
– swabs taken from ears, nose, throat etc.
– information pack given to parents

It is useful to give relatives a copy of *What to do after a death*,[3] a Department of Social Security booklet. When they are ready to leave A&E, a contact name and telephone number of the A&E department should be given, to enable any subsequent questions to be dealt with. Any written information given to relatives should be recorded.

As always, make sure that the name of the doctor and nurse dealing with the relatives and death of the patient are clearly legible.

Patients' property

If patients' property has had to be cut or is grossly soiled it is unlikely the relatives will want to take it home, but they should not be denied the opportunity. All property, irrespective of the condition, should be listed in the property book which must be completed as scrupulously as any other nursing record and labelled with the patient's identification details. The next of kin will be required to sign for receipt of any of the patient's belongings.

Detail who has received the property in the patient's notes to enable subsequent enquiries to be dealt with sensitively and efficiently.

On occasion, following a serious assault or murder the police will request to receive all of the patient's clothing. This needs to be documented in exactly the same way, using the property book but obviously it is the policeman who signs for receipt.

Attention to detail when making records allows the individual making that record to recall the patient at a later date. Clarity and logical sequences of the A&E notes allows another reader to move swiftly through the information to the pertinent area e.g.

'A nurse manager is following up a claim to a lost ring which the patient says, was removed in the accident department one month ago. According to the A&E record card, NO mention of the ring is made.'

Less than 20 seconds are needed to add this information:

'Yellow metal ring, cut and returned to patient. 1650 hrs.

I.S. Clear

The nurse can ask the patient to sign the A&E card or similarly ask a colleague to witness the return of the ring. This 20 seconds of information saves time for the patient, manager, and nurse when the claim was followed up.

Telephone advice

One's responsibility towards a patient starts at the first contact and this does not need to be at a face to face meeting. For this reason all enquiries and advice by telephone must be documented in a structured way. (Ideally all A&E departments should have a telephone system that records conversations.)

For patients who have previously attended the A&E department whose enquiry is regarding their current injury, the problem and advice can be written on the A&E notes e.g.

'23/6/94. 1300 hrs.
Pt discharged two days ago. Now complaining of increased swelling and pain over wound site. Dressing intact. ADVICE: Simple analgesia, elevation and to either return to A&E or see GP if problem continues over next 12/24 hrs.'

Signed: *A. Cist*

Other enquiries and advice given for patient problems should be documented in a book (not loose leaf). When making an entry it is advisable (where possible), to record the patient's name and if appropriate their age. All enquiries should be signed and dated and the time of the call should be added e.g.

3/6/94. 0715 hrs.
'3-year-old possibly ingested 2 × 50 mcg. Thyroxine tabs less than one hour ago. Tel—Mrs Brown 940 518.
Poisons Centre contacted Recommend that no treatment is required unless over 125 mcg. To attend if any symptoms. Advice offered as above—Mrs Brown will attend if worried.'

Signed: *C. Pills*

It is not unusual to receive an enquiry form an anonymous called. 'A friend of mine has just taken 10 paracetamol. Is it dangerous?' It can be difficult to obtain any details from someone who is reluctant to give the information. However, you might be told the friend's age and even if this is all the information you have it is still essential to document the call e.g.

10/3/94. 2000 hrs.
Male caller. friend 18 years old. (no name offered) taken 10 paracetamol <1 hour ago.
ADVICE: Encouraged to bring friend to hospital. If no transport—advised to phone for any ambulance.

Signed: *E. Scape*

People telephone for advice and on all sorts of health-related problems. Although one can use one's experience to answer questions asked, we cannot see the patient and do not have access to their medical records. Do not diagnose over the telephone.

A diagnosis made over the telephone is akin to determining whether or not the patient is cyanotic in a completely dark room. Jean Balsama Dunn[4]

Effective communication is the stepping stone between each stage, of treatment for the patient and between colleagues. If it happens, has been said, or done—write it down. Remember that once it is written down it becomes a part of a legal document and although the spoken word is often forgotten the written word *cannot* be forgotten.

References

1. United Kingdom Central Council (UKCC) (1993). *Standards for records and record keeping*, pp. 15–16, April.
2. Smith, I. (1989). Waterlow/Norton Scoring System—A ward view. *Care—Science and Practice*, **7**(4), 93–5.
3. Department of Social Security. (1993). *What to do after a death*. Leaflet D49. HMSO, London.
4. Dunn, J. B. (1988). Legal considerations and documentation. In *Handbook of emergency nursing—The nursing process approach*, (ed. L. Mowad and D. C. Ruhle), pp. 9–16. Appleton & Lange, Norwalk, Conn., USA.

Index